Stress Management and Your Health

Stress Management and Your Health

Joseph Nii Abekar Mensah, PhD.

Clinical/Educational Consultant.
Progressive Learning Institute & Counselling Services,
Calgary, Alberta, Canada.

Strategic Book Publishing and Rights Co.

Copyright © 2013 by Joseph Nii Abekar Mensah, PhD..
All rights reserved.

No part of this book may be reproduced or transmitted in any form or by any means, electronic or mechanical, including photocopy, recording or any information storage and retrieval system, without prior written permission from the author.

Strategic Book Publishing and Rights Co.
12620 FM 1960, Suite A4-507
Houston TX 77065
www.sbpra.com

ISBN 978-1-62212-585-2

Dedication

This book is dedicated to the loving memories of my deceased sisters who passed away in their flowers of youth namely, Naa Tettehley (fio), Naa Jama, Naa Aba, and my late brother, Emma; and my nieces: Elsie Marbell, and Lola Marbell. You are all dearly loved and missed. Rest in Peace. It is also dedicated to the fondest memories of my late father, Nii Larbi Mensah II (Atofo Mantse, Nii Sempe Mensa We), my late mother, Mary Naa Addoley-Okailey Addo; my loving grandparents, Nii Abeka "Sikafo" (Nii Sempe Mensa We), Naa Fofo, Naa Klorkai Hammond (Osu, Kinkawe), Nii Adote Addo, and the rest of my immediate, the extended family, too numerous to mention individually.

Acknowledgements

The author gives thank to God in Jesus Name for the love and blessings HE has bestowed upon me throughout my life. Most importantly, I give thanks and praises to the Almighty for giving me wisdom, inspiration and guidance as I write this book.

A word of thanks and appreciation to members of my immediate and extended family, especially Victoria Naa Koshi Lamptey, Mrs. Adelaide Naa Addoley Marbell, Nii John Vanderpuye, Theresa Naa Darkua Dodoo (Osu Manye), Professor Nii Ablorh Odijah and Joseph Nii Ankonu Annan, who have been pillars of encouragement to me, personally, and in my writing efforts.

Thanks also to Dr. Ellis Quarshie and Mr. Michael Quarshie, whose friendship, love and inspiration to me are extremely well appreciated, and which will forever linger in my mind.

Also, many thanks and appreciation to Patricia Brown for her painstaking efforts in typing part of this book. Special word of thanks and appreciation to my son, Ebenezer Nii Sempeh Mensah, for his love and support, and for coping with a preoccupied father as I write this book.

TABLE OF CONTENTS

PREFACE xiii

CHAPTER ONE

Introduction 1

    Underlying Mechanism of Stress 8
    Fight or Flight Response 9
    Mobilization of the Body 9
    G.A.S and Burnout 10
    Thought Processes and Stress 11
    Integrated Stress Response 12
    How Stress Affects Your Health 12
    Diseases Caused By Stress 12
    Stress and Immune Diseases 14
    Stress and the Risk of Heart Attack 14
    Stress and Personality 16
    Key Characteristics of Type A Personality 18
    Techniques of Managing Stress 19
    References 21

CHAPTER TWO
Systematic Treatment of Causes of Stress 22

    Physiological Theories of Stress 24
    Psychological Theories of Stress 33
    Environmental Theories of Stress 40
    Summary 44
    References 46

CHAPTER THREE
Manifestations and Effects of Stress 49

    Multiple Effects 56
    Effects of Stress 60
    Depression 63
    Lowered Effectiveness and Efficiency 66
    Summary 67
    References 70

CHAPTER FOUR
Stress Management and Counseling 71

    Coping Mechanisms 71
    Relaxation and Meditation 77
    Relaxation and Cycle Breaking 78
    Body Therapy 81
    Psychological Therapies 88
    Coping Mechanisms and the Physiological Causes of Stress 94

Summary	96
Reference	97

CHAPTER FIVE
Stress Management Techniques in Other Cultures and Religion	99
Hinduism	99
Buddhism	101
Christianity	102
Islam	103
Jainism	104
Judaism	104
New Age Meditation	105
Sikhism	105
Taoism	105
Bahai Faith	106
Active Dynamic Meditation	106
Health Applications of Meditation	107
References	108

BIBLIOGRAPHY   111

PREFACE

Stress is a threat to the quality of life and to the physical and psychological well being: that is the premise of this book. Should this be the case, every effort must be made to understand its nature, its causes, and its manifestations, and the different ways in which we can effectively manage or cope with stress.

I have experienced extremely stressful situations or circumstances these past few years of my life. In an attempt to cope with my stressors and the negative impact they may have on my physical and psychological well being I relied on my faith in God, believing that God will not let anything come my way that He knows I cannot handle. I also resorted to reading a thesis I had written about thirty one years ago. These along with other stress management techniques I read by different authors and researchers, have helped me a great deal to cope with my own situation successfully. Thus, I thought I should revisit my earlier studies and share my thoughts on the subject with the wider public. Hopefully, this study may help someone.

Stress has been studied by many investigators, and from different points of view. However, there is still a need for an integrated study which can introduce many of these view points and relate one to another. This book examines stress at the level of the individual, discussing it as a personal phenomenon. It also treats stress as a problem of all types of society.

The book presents the topic stress in two ways. Firstly, the book attempts to ensure that some commonly quoted statements about stress are explained. By so doing, it would provide a comprehensive and rather detailed introduction to the subject. Secondly, it takes these discussions further by examining specific topics in some detail.

In chapter one, the different approaches to the interpretation and analysis of stress are examined. This section also provides a framework for this book. In Chapter Two, the relationship between the concepts of stress and passion is examined. The experience of stress is put into the context of the general understanding of emotion, and the neural mechanisms involved in the control of that experience are outlined. Here, the author also examines in detail the theories of stress and their implications for counseling, relying heavily on the work of Hans Selye, Cannon and many other leading investigators in the field. The causes and manifestations of stress, responses to stress are described in Chapter Three. This is divided first into physiological, psychological and environmental components and are broken down into their many and varied aspects. In the Fourth Chapter, the writer has examined the various coping mechanisms to stress and has concluded that there is no panacea for stress. People under stress may resort to alcohol, smoking, tranquilizers, sedatives and narcotics as means of coping. Biofeedback, meditation, and relaxation techniques are explored. Other stress management techniques explored in this chapter include body therapy, structural integration, etc. Psychological therapies examined include Transactional Analysis by Berne, Rational Emotive Therapy proposed by Dr. Albert Ellis, Reality Therapy propounded by William Glaser and Assertive Therapy. This book attempts to bring them together into a general framework. The relationship between psychopharmacology and stress management has also been considered. Finally, in Chapter Five, the author has discussed the management of stress cross-culturally, and in other religions, such as Hinduism, Buddhism, Christianity, Islam, Jainism, Judaism, Sikhism, Taoism, Bahai Faith, and Krishnamurti idea of meditation. Health applications of meditation have been given some attention.

In general, this book makes reference to pharmacology, physiology and biochemistry, psychiatry and psychology, community health and a full range of other bio-medical and social sciences. Because it is an integrated study, it may help bridge the gap between many of these disciplines in the study of stress.

Readers of this book should bear in mind that stress can cause serious health problems and in extreme cases, can cause death. While these stress management techniques referred to in this book have been shown to have positive effect on reducing stress, they are for guidance only. Thus, readers of this book are strongly advised to seek the opinion of a duly qualified and/or certified mental health professionals or physicians if they have any concerns over stress-related illness or if stress is causing serious or chronic pain. Health professionals should also be consulted before any major change in diet or levels of exercise.

The author hopes that this book will be easily readable by a wide range of readers. The content of this book cross many different disciplines, and it may be, hopefully, applicable to individuals, the academic community, many different professions, and for the informed and interested layperson.

The author must finally declare that the responsibility for any errors, omissions and opinions expressed are solely his.

CHAPTER ONE

INTRODUCTION

Stress is a threat to the quality of life, and to physical and psychological well-being: that is the premise of this book. Stress has been likened to a dangerous virus that has infected modern man. We have all noted its symptoms, the knot of tension in one's stomach. The splitting headache caused by the pressures of life. The feeling that one is going to explode, that one just cannot take it anymore.

Dubbed the "Twentieth Century Killer", stress arises primarily from the Psychological demands of life. The effects of stress on the body can be extremely serious. Should we personally be concerned about it, for ourselves as well as one's family? It is the author's belief that the answer is yes. Stress is linked to physical illness. Research has shown that intense or prolonged stress can make the body more vulnerable to ailments ranging from skin rashes and the common cold to heart attacks and cancer. It is believed that the epidemic of stress, with its resulting damage, affects only adults in particular high-pressure jobs. If that were so, why would Dr. Coley had said that stress affects all of us? Stress today afflicts both young and old, including many persons who we might not think would be affected.

The concept of stress is ambiguous because it is poorly defined. There is no single agreed definition in existence. It is a concept which is familiar to both layman and professional alike. "Stress" means different things to different people. The term conveys to many the thought of tension or pressure. This is only part or the picture.

In newspaper accounts of some airplanes crashes, one may have read that stress lead to metal fatigue, causing a part to fail, and the plane to crash. That stress was a force on a piece of metal that tended to damage or distort it. It snapped. The plane crashed.

In some ways, it can be comparable with human stress. It is some physical or emotional issue that affects the body, to which we need to adjust or else we may be harmed. It is common to think of stress in connection with emotional strain or stress, which can cause physical changes. When we do not comprehend what changes are occurring in us, one may not know how to cooperate with one's body's attempt to adapt. While physically and emotionally one may be equipped to recover from stress, the effects of stress tend to be cumulative. Complicating this is the fact that as one ages (perhaps speeded up by stress itself) one's ability to respond to stress diminishes.

Hans Selye has pointed out that many factors affect one's reaction to stress. These include physiological predispositions, early childhood experiences, personality, and social resources. Kobasa et al (1979) suggested that specific aspects of personality interact with specific aspects of the social conditions in many ways, leading to more or less resilience. For that reason, researchers need to know a terrific deal more about the expectations and social pressures within different groups.

Kobasa explained that the process whereby stressful life events cause disease is undoubtedly physiological. Whatever this physiological response is, the personality characteristics of "hardiness" may cut into its decreasing the likelihood of breakdown into illness.

Hans Selye has argued that certain kinds of stress which he calls "eu-stress" are good for people. Selye has described the body's actual response to stress in several experiments. Since then, he has pointed out that the racing pulse, the quickened heart rate that betrays stress also occur during the time of massive job. A certain amount of stress is essential to well-being, through people requirements will vary. Selye suggested that there are two main types of human beings: "race horses" that are only satisfied with a vigorous, fast-paced lifestyle, and "turtles" that want peace, quiet, and tranquil environment". The trick is to find the amount of stress that best suits the individual.

Dr. Robert Ader contends that a feeling of helplessness would be one of the psychological factors which could trigger disease. He maintains that conditions are optimal for a physical breakdown, where there is a biological predisposition. Stress is an inability to cope with stressors. He argues that in a healthy individual, there is a balance or coordination among these forces but that there is an unusually high biological predisposition to a particular disease. It takes remarkably little stress to disrupt this inner harmony and accelerate the disease. From this, it follows that someone less vulnerable would require a much larger portion of stress before developing the same disease.

Stress affects people of all ages, and people in different types of occupations. However, dozens of studies in the past three decades have shown that people who are in high-stress occupations or who have suffered a serious setback in their lives run an unusually high risk of disease. However, such disease is not inevitable, despite the increased risk. Researchers in the area of stress are now emphasizing that large numbers of people do not get ill under stress.

Thus, many people work night and day at vigorous jobs without becoming ill while others who have seemingly easier occupations develop ulcers, hypertension or heart disease. Some people survive even the horrors of a concentration camp; while others cannot cope with everyday problems without falling apart, mentally or physically.

The question as to why some people stay healthy is one of the most intriguing questions in medical science today. Aged and heredity surely help. Investigators in the field of behavioral treatment are only starting to learn how different kinds of behavior, such as the restless striving and frustration of so-called Type A's, are related to such disease as hypertension or coronary disease. Though research is still in its infancy, we now have a few clues to the physiological qualities and social environment that may account for resilience to stress.

Kobasa, et al (1979) defined some of the characteristics of what they call "hardiness". They suggest that stress-resistant people have a specific set of attitudes toward life, and are opens to change. They have a sense of control of events. In the jargon of psychological research, they soar high on "challenge" (viewing change as a challenge rather than a threat), "commitment" (the opposite of alienation) and "control" (the opposite of powerlessness). These attitudes have a profound effect on health, according to the Kobosa and associate, who have been studying the prevalence of life stresses, and illness among hundreds of business executives, lawyers, military officials and elderly people.

This book identifies the stressors in one's daily life, and suggests corrective and/or counseling approach to combating stress; and thereby maintaining good health. The book is prompted by concerns of the author; problems of some of his family and co-workers most of whom are in the teaching, and the helping professions, and who expressed their inability to cope with the stressors in their daily lives.

However, this book suffers the following limitations. Though ample literature on stress is available there has not been a previous attempt to understand the stressors and their relationships to autoimmune disease.

Much of information about the effects of stress in the existing research literature is still fragmentary-or even contradictory. Depending on circumstances, for example, anxiety can get one's heart beat either faster or slower (as when the heart "stands still"). Even more surprisingly, some kinds of stress will cause breast cancers develop in mice, but the same stress will slow down or actually inhibit the spread of breast cancers in rats. Eventually, with more research, we may be able to alleviate some of the dangerous effects of stress.

The book is based primarily on literature review, which as mentioned earlier, the information is still sketchy or even contradictory.

This book fails to distinguish the stressors (if any) in the various aspects on the individual and of the professions, such as nursing and the teaching professions, such as the stressors experienced by the nurse in the intensive care unit as opposed to the stressors experienced by the nurse working in the pediatric care unit, and elementary school teacher, as opposed to the junior high or the high school teacher, for example.

The book examines the theories of stress and the effects of stress on the body; and its impacts on autoimmune diseases. The stressors would be examined in detail. Counseling and other therapeutic models are prescribed to help people to achieve the stressors they encounter in everyday life.

The problems of stress are multifaceted. It is not easy to determine one particular set of causative factors which could be defined as being the root of the problem. Certain stressful circumstances are influenced through the process of counseling and/or therapy. It seemed necessary to touch on some of the most theoretical basis of stress and the harmful effects of stress.

The author deals with needs and values, the ever changing society, which leads to stress. The role of counseling in preparing professions as well as the general public in dealing with stress is not a new and unique idea. It is somewhat controversial. The points discussed in this book do not contradict the significant social and economic demands on individuals and their families, which may lead to stress, depression and severe mental ailments. Not uncommonly, the professions have chosen to view stressors and their associated problems through counseling, training or rehabilitative strategies, rather than attack the roots of the problem. Furthermore, it would be impossible within the confines of this book to give in-depth analysis of each of the biological, physiological, environmental, personality, early childhood experiences and psychosocial issues, which are directly implicated with stress.

The book is based upon the following assumptions. Stress and how to deal with it is increasingly becoming problem of serious concern to the professions and in society generally. Any significant change is stressful. Counseling and/or therapy-including the development of specific programs for the individual may lead to something better in the lives of those participating.

Stress is a condition or feeling experienced when a person perceives that demands exceed the physical and social resources the individual is able to muster. Distress and stress are words commonly used in connection with the word stress.

Indeed it is possible that they share the same root. One may explain distress as a severe strain of pain, or sorrow, and anguish, exhaustion or breathlessness. Attention is given to the exertion required to meet demands, damage or replacement resulting from the condition of a body subjected to stress.

Fatigue, another term commonly used in the same context as stress is defined as weariness after exertion or prolonged strain. Although studying the origins, meanings and shared use of words rarely solves problems of precise definition, in this particular case it provides a definite starting point for an attempt at that solution. Implicit in these definitions is a kind of stress which is regarded as a constraining force on a person. In attempting to cope with this force the person feels fatigued and distressed.

A cursory survey of the available scientific literature reveals that studies on stress can be easily placed into one of three groups representing the main approaches to the question of its definition. Lazarus (1966), Appley and Trumbell (1967), McGrath (1970) have discussed these approaches in some detail, and the main points raised in those discussions will be dealt with briefly in this book. The first approach treats stress as a dependent variable for analysis, describing it in terms of the body's response to disturbing or harmful environments. The following method describes stress in terms of the stimulus characteristics of those disturbing or harmful environments; which usually treats it as an independent variable for analysis. The third and perhaps most reasonable means views stress, as the reflection of a "lack of consistency" between the individual and his environment. Stress in this form is studied in terms of its antecedent factors and its effects. It is seen as an intervening variable between stimulus and response. There is common ground between these different approaches, and they differ most in where they put the value in the definitions they offer, and in the methods they adopt.

In all three approaches, the word environment, is used in the widest sense, and refers to both the body's internal and external environments, as well as his physical and psychosocial environments. In short, stress may be defined as a complex condition of body and brain caused by abnormal or threatening situations in the external world, and persisting until these situations are removed. The condition may be short or long term, and the causes or stressors may be either physiological or psychological, with the latter tending to be more problematic. All human beings, from birth to death, are subject to occasional bursts of stress. Stress is conceptualized as a universal phenomenon in which the individual perceives environmental stimuli as taxing the physiological or social systems, whereby responses can be adaptive or maladaptive. This interpretation is supported to some degree by the work of two eminent researchers.

The author has borrowed heavily on the work of Dr. Hans Selye, the father of the "stress theory", and the creation of Dr. Richard Lazarus, who has been concerned with the psychological aspects of stress. Selye has defined stress in physiological terms as "the nonspecific responses of the body to any demands made upon it" (Selye 1975). Lazarus has defined stress as environmental, of internal demands that stress or exceed the adaptive resources of a system (Lazarus, 1971).

Both Selye and Lazarus emphasize the importance of perception in determining whether or not a stressor is negative or positive. Perception is a psychological phenomenon. It involves receiving information and the cognitive appraisal of that information. In cognitive appraisal, phenomena are categorized as to their positive or adverse effects on human beings. Uncertainty about the nature of a stimulus encourages arousal of the protective physiological mechanisms of the body. Individuals react as if they were under threat. This may or may not, in reality, be justifiable. If individuals react to a stimulus; and if it is threatening and, in actuality, it is not, then mentally they must maintain their cognitive stability by rationalizing their defensive behavior (Festinger, 1957; Heider, 1958).

Sometimes this behavior leads to long chains of rationalization and overt actions that culminate in actual psychological and physiological decrease.

Underlying Mechanism of Stress

There are two types of instinctive stress response that are relevant to how we understand the stress and stress management: the short-term "Fight-Flight response and the long-term "General Adaptation Syndrome". The first is basic survival instinct. The second is a long-term result to stress. The third mechanism comes from the way that we think and understand the situations in which we find ourselves. These three mechanisms can be part of the same stress response. Let us initially review them separately, and then determine how they can join together.

Fight-or-Flight Response:

Some of the early work on stress conducted by Walter Cannon (1932) established the existence of the well-known "fight-or-flight" response. Cannon's observation showed that when an animal experiences a shock or perceives a threat, it immediately releases hormones that support it to survive. These hormones help us to run faster and fight harder. They increase heart rate and blood pressure, delivering more oxygen and blood sugar to power important muscles. This result in increase sweating in an effort to cool these muscles, and help them stay efficiently. They divert blood away from the skin to the core of one's body, reducing blood loss if the body is damaged. At the same time, one's attention is focused on these hormones and the risk that confronts us, to the exclusion of everything else. All of this significantly improves one's ability to survive life-threatening events.

Mobilization of the Body

Unfortunately, this mobilization of the body for survival also has negative consequences. In this state, we are excitable, anxious, jumpy, and irritable. This reduces the person's ability to work effectively with other people. With trembling and a pounding heart, we think it difficult to execute precise, controlled skills. The intensity of one's attention on survival interferes with his or her capability for real judgments based on drawing information from various sources. As a result, we find ourselves more accident-prone and less able to make good decisions. It is easy to think that this fight-or-flight or adrenaline (epinephrine) reaction is caused by unpleasant life-threatening danger. On the contrary, recent research shows that we meet the fight-or-flight response when clearly encountering something unexpected.

The situation does not have to be dramatic. People experience this response when frustrated or interrupted, or when they encounter a situation that is new or in some way challenging. This hormonal, fight-or-flight response is a normal part of everyday life and part of everyday stress, although often with an intensity that is so small that we do not see. There are remarkably few situations in modern working life where this response is helpful. Most situations benefit from a calm, rational, controlled and socially sensitive approach. Relaxation techniques are useful for keeping this fight-or-flight reaction under control.

The General Adaptation Syndrome and Burnout

Hans Selye took a different approach from Cannon. Starting with the observation that different diseases and injuries to the body, seemed to generate the same symptoms in patients, Selye identified a typical reaction (the "General Adaptation Syndrome") with which the body reacts to a major stimulus. While the fight-or-flight response works in the very short-term, the General Adaptation Syndrome operates in response to longer-term exposure to causes of stress.

Selye identified that when pushed to the extreme, animals reacted to three signals. First, in the Alarm Phase, they reacted to the stressor. Next, in the Resistance Phase, the response to the stressor increased as the animal adapted to, and coped with it. This phase lasted for as long as the animal could keep this heightened resistance. Finally, once one's response is exhausted, the individual enters the Exhaustion Phase, the resistance declines significantly.

In today's business environment, the fatigue is seen in "burnout". The perfect example comes from the Wall Street trading floor.

Burnout

Burnout is characterized by a significantly reduced energy level. The individual may suffer from feelings of alienation as evidenced by withdrawing from work and other groups and interests. There is a tendency to show negative feelings towards others, characterized by negative and defamatory remarks. The person may also begin to distrust and blame others. Burnout appears to be a factor in lowered morale, absenteeism, and lowered work performance as well as physical signs and symptoms of illness.

Thought Processes and Stress

In a particular working situation, much of one's stress is subtle and occurs without apparent threat to the survival. Most comes from things like work overload, conflicting priorities, inconsistent values, one's demanding deadlines, and conflicts with co-workers, unfriendly environments and so on. Not only do these lower body's performance as one diverts mental energy into handling them, they can also create a considerable amount of unhappiness.

As indicated earlier, the most popular currently accepted definition of stress is something that is experienced when a person perceives demands as exceeding one's personal and social resources one is able to assemble. In becoming stressed one must make two main judgments. In the first

place, one must feel threatened by the situation, and secondly one must suspect that one's capabilities and resources are sufficient to meet the threat.

How stressed the person feels depends on how much damage he or she thinks the situation can make him or her, and how his or her resources meet the demands of the situation. This sense of danger is rarely visible. It may, for example, include perceived threats to one's social status, to other people's opinion of us, to our career prospects, or to our own deeply held values. Just as with real threats to individual's survival, these perceived threats trigger the hormonal fight-or-flight response, with all its negative consequences.

The Integrated Stress Response

So far, the author has presented the Fight-or Flight response, the General Adaptation Syndrome, and the individual's psychological response to stress as separate mechanisms. As a matter of fact, both the Fight-or-Flight response and the General Adaptation Syndrome can fit together into one response. The key to this is that Hans Selye's "Alarm Phase" is the same thing as Walter Cannon's Fight-or Flight response.

From the foregoing, it seems clear that mental stress triggers the "fight-or-flight" response; and that if this stress is sustained for a long time, the result must be exhaustion and burnout.

HOW STRESS AFFECTS YOUR HEALTH
Diseases Caused By Stress

Perhaps, we may raise the question as to what diseases are caused by stress; and what are the mechanisms by which stress causes these diseases. The effects of stress on one's body have far reaching impact on each of every system of the body. The conversion of emotional distress to physiological change, and hence to a physical manifestation is known as" transduction"; a situation is perceived, a value is assigned to it, an emotional response is elicited, and a physiological reaction results. Complex autoimmune, hormonal and neuromuscular mechanisms mediate this response. This may itself affect the environment, generating in turn a social response that may generate a positive or negative feedback.

Somatization, or alteration of emotional distress into physical illness, is an extremely fundamental concept that recognizes that an emotionally distressed being more often presents with physical symptoms than psychological complaints. Experts believe that people who somatize are alexithymic. This implies that such people cannot express their feelings in words and must, therefore, resort to expressing them in real symptoms. Some of the diseases that are induced, sustained or exacerbated by stress include: 1) Acid Peptic Disease; 2) Alcoholism; 3) Asthma; 4) Fatigue; 5) Hypertension; 6) Insomnia; 7) Irritable Bowel Syndrome; 8) Tension Headache; 9) Ischemic Heart Disease; 10) Psychoneurosis; 11) Sexual Dysfunction; 12) Skin Diseases like psoriasis, neuro dermatitis, and so forth.

Many of the effects of stress on the mind and body are due to increased sympathetic nervous system activity and an outpouring of adrenaline (epinephrine), cortisol and other stress-related hormones. Certain types of chronic and more subtle stress due to abandonment, poverty, bereavement, despair and irritation due to discrimination are associated with impaired immune system resistance to viral linked disorders ranging from the common cold and herpes to AIDS and cancer.

Stress can have effects on other hormones, brain neurotransmitters, another tiny chemical messengers elsewhere, prostaglandins, as well as critical enzyme systems, and metabolic activities. Research in these areas may help to explain how stress can contribute to depression, anxiety and its adverse effects on the gastrointestinal tract, skin and other organs. Understanding the above concepts are extremely vital in understanding the diseases caused by stress and to create a plan of action for the management of stress and stress induced diseases.

Stress and Autoimmune Diseases

Medical scientists believe that the etiology of autoimmune diseases is multifactorial: genetic, environmental, hormonal, and immunological factors are all considered valuable in their development. Nevertheless, the onset of at least fifty percent of autoimmune disorders has been attributed to "unknown trigger factors. Physical and emotional stress has been implicated in the development of autoimmune diseases. Numerous animal and human studies have demonstrated the effects of various stressors on immune function. Moreover, several retrospective studies

found that a high proportion (up to 80 percent) of patients reported remarkable emotional stress before illness onset.

Unfortunately, not only does stress cause diseases, but the disease itself also causes significant stress in the patients, creating a vicious cycle. Recent reviews explore the potential role of psychological stress, and of the greatest stress-related hormones, in the pathogenesis of autoimmune disease. It is presumed that the stress-triggered neuroendocrine hormones lead to immune deregulation, which ultimately results in autoimmune disease by altering or amplifying cytokine production. Thus, the treatment of autoimmune disease should include stress management and behavioral intervention to prevent stress-related immune imbalance. Physicians and clinical psychologists should examine different reactions with their autoimmune patients, and unavoidable questionnaire about trigger factors should include emotional stress in addition to inflammation, pain and other common triggers.

Stress and Risk of Heart Attack

The question is whether there is a relationship between stress and risk of heart attack. Does stress increase the risk of heart disease? Stress is a normal part of life. However, if left uncontrolled or managed, stress can lead to emotional, psychological, and even physical problems, including heart disease, chest pain or irregular heart beats. Medical researchers are not entirely sure as to how stress increases the risk of heart disease. Stress itself might be a risk factor, or it could be that high levels of stress make other risk factors, such as hypertension, worse. For example, if a person is under stress, his or her blood pressure goes up, he/she may over eat, or may eat less, and he/she is more likely to smoke.

If stress itself is a risk factor for heart disease, it could be because chronic stress exposes the body to harmful, persistently elevated levels of stress hormones like adrenaline (epinephrine) and cortisol. Studies also link stress to changes in the way blood clots, which increases the risk. People react differently to events and situations. One person may perceive an event joyful and gratifying. Another person may find the same event miserable and frustrating. Sometimes, people may feel stress in ways that produce unpleasant situations worse by reacting with feelings

of anger, guilt, fear, hostility, and moodiness, while others may experience life's challenges with ease.

Stress can be caused by physical or emotional changes in the environment that requires a person to alter or respond. Things that make one feel stressed are known as stressors. Stressors can be lesser hassles, significant lifestyle changes, or a combination of both. Being able to identify stressors in one's life and releasing the anxiety they produce are the keys to managing stress. The following are some common stressors that can affect us at different stages of life. 1) Illness either of a family member or a friend. 2) Death of a friend or loved one. 3) Work overload. 4) Starting a new job. 5) Unemployment. 6) Pregnancy. 7) Crowds. 8) Relocation. 9) Daily. 10) Hassles. 10) Legal problems. 11) Financial concerns. 12) Perfectionism

When one is exposed to a long period of stress, the body gives warning signals that something is wrong. These physical, cognitive, emotional and behavioral warning signs should not be ignored. They tell us we need to slow down. If the individual continues to be stressed, and fails to provide his/her body a chance, he/she is likely to develop health problems and heart disease. The following is some of the common signs and symptoms of stress.

Physical Signs

Dizziness, general aches and pains, grinding teeth, clenched jaws, indigestion, muscle tension, difficulty sleeping, racing heart, ringing in the ears, stooped posture, sweaty palms, tiredness, exhaustion, trembling, weight gain or loss, and upset stomach.

Mental Signs

Constant worry, difficulty making decisions, forgetfulness, inability to concentrate, lack of creativity, loss of sense of humor, and poor memory.

Emotional Signs

Anger, anxiety, crying, depression, feeling of powerlessness, frequent mood swings, irritability, loneliness, negative thinking, nervousness, and sadness.

Behavioral Signs

Bussiness, compulsive eating, critical thinking of others, explosive actions, frequent job changes, impulsive actions, increased use of alcohol or drugs, withdrawal from relationships or social situations.

Stress and Personality Types

What is stressful to one person may not be stress to another person. The difference appears to be in one's perceptions of different events. Mental health professionals believe personality plays a significant role in how the individual perceives stress. People with "Type A" personalities, for example, are rushed, ambitious, time conscious and driven. Studies suggest these traits if not properly managed, can make stress-related illness. In contrast, the "Type B" personality is much more relaxed, less time conscious and driven individual. Type B personalities are able to see things more adaptively. They are better able to put things into perspective, and think through how they are going to deal with situations. Conversely, they tend to be less stress-prone.

The Development of Personality Type

The question is what causes these differences in personalities. A various social, biological, emotional and behavior factors influence the development one's character. Scientists agree that a largely genetic physical chemistry, or in-born temperament, influences a baby to respond to his or her environment in ways that can be assertive or shy. Such tendencies are also influenced by one's experiences. The combination of heritage and experience from an individual's way of behaving, feeling and thinking make up his personality.

Also, studies show that men and women handle stress differently; a difference that some researchers attribute, in part, to estrogen. The hormonal differences may also account for the fact that women are three times more likely to develop depression in response to the stressors in their lives than are men. Women, unlike men, also tend to have stronger social support networks to which they turn during times of stress. These social supports may help explain why women, in general, seem to be better able to cope with stress than men.

Impact of Early Experiences on Stress Response

Research suggests that person's response to stress could be influence by one's experience in the womb. Scientists have been studying mechanisms by which maternal stress, and the resulting high levels of cortisol in her body during pregnancy, could affect the development of the baby. Researcher believe that if the mother has high levels of cortisol, the fetus will have similar high level of receptors for stress-related substances in the brain which may make them more susceptible to stressors later in life. Even after birth, a mother's response to stress affects her baby. If a mother is stressed or depressed during the early years of her child's life, she may not create a good relationship with her child. Worse, there could be long-term consequences on the child's stress response, behavior and intelligence.

Even people with most versatile personalities can experience the effects of long-term stress if they lack a sense of control over aspects of their daily lives. Scientists believe that people who have the least control over their working environment suffer from higher level of stress-related illnesses.

Key Traits or characteristics of "Type A" Personality

Even though, the term "Type A" is thrown around often, it is not always fully known what specific character "Type A" Personality, even among the experts. For example, for some people, the term applies to harsh and anxious people. Others see workaholics as "Type A" Many see competitiveness as the main characteristics. Researchers believe that the following characteristics are the hallmark characteristics of "Type "behavior.

Time Urgency and Impatience, as demonstrated by people, who, among other things, get frustrated, while waiting in line, interrupts others often, walk or talk at a rapid pace, and are always painfully aware of the time and short of it they have to spare.

Another Type behavior includes: Competitiveness; Higher Achievement Motivation; Certain Physical Characteristics that results from stress are Facial Tension (Tight Lips, Clenched Jaw; Dark circles under eyes; Facial Sweating.

Negative Effects of Type A Behavior.

Over the years, the kind of extra stress that most Type A person's experience take a toll on their health and lifestyle. The following are some of the negative effects that are ordinary individuals with Type A personality. These include hypertension and heart diseases.

Techniques for Managing Stress

After one has identified the causes of stress in one's life, the next step is to learn techniques that may help one to cope. There are many techniques one can use to manage stress. Some of which the individual can learn by himself/herself while other techniques may require the guidance of a trained therapist. Some techniques for coping with stress include:

Eat and drink sensibly. Abusing alcohol and food may seem to reduce stress, but it actually adds to it.

Assert yourself: One does not have to meet other's expectations or demands. It is OK to say "no". Being assertive allows one to stand for the individual's rights and beliefs, while respecting those of others.

Do not Smoke: Aside from the obvious health risks of cigarettes, nicotine acts as a stimulant and brings on more stress symptoms.

Exercise: Choose a non-competitive task and set realistic goals. Aerobic exercise releases endorphins (neutral substance that help the individual feel better and maintain a positive attitude).

Relax every day: Choose from a variety of different techniques. I will discuss this in details later in this book.

Reduce the Causes of Stress: Many people think life filled with too many demands and too little time. For the most part, those demands are ones we have chosen. Effective time-management skills involve asking for help when appropriate, setting priorities, pacing one's self, and taking time out for oneself.

One must examine one's values and live by them: The more one's actions reflect one's beliefs, the better one will notice, no matter how busy one is.

Set Realistic Goals and Expectations: It is OK and beneficial to realize that one cannot be 100 percent successful at everything all at once.

Sell oneself to oneself: When we are feeling overwhelmed, one must try maintaining a healthy sense of self-esteem.

Get Enough Rest: Even with proper diet and exercise, one cannot fight stress effectively without rest. One needs time to recover from exercise and stressful events. The time one spends resting should be long enough to relax one's mind as well as one's body. Some people think that taking a nap in the middle of the day helps them reduce stress.

A positive attitude and self-esteem are good defenses against stress and heart diseases. This is because they help us to see stress as a challenge rather than a problem. A positive attitude keeps the person in control when there are certain changes in one's life. A positive attitude means telling oneself there are things one can do to improve certain situations and admitting sometimes there's nothing one can do. To maintain a positive attitude during a stressful situation, one must keep these tips in mind.

11) Stay Calm: Stop what one is doing. Breathe deeply. Reflect on one's choices. Believe that one can go through the situation. Try to be objective, practical and versatile. Try to keep the situation in perspective. Think about the possible solutions. Choose one that is the most satisfying and adaptable.

Think about the outcome. Ask one, what is the worst possible thing that can happen? Tell one that one can learn something from every situation.

References

1. Selye, Hans. *The Stress of Life.* New York: McGraw-Hill Book Company, 1956
2. Selye, Hans, *Stress.* Montreal: Acta, 1950
3. Kobasa, Suzanne et al., *Journal of Occupational Medicine,* 21(1979):595-8.
4. Selye Hans, On the Real Benefits of Eustress", *Psychology Today,* March, 1978.
5. Broadbent, D.E. *Decision and Stress,* London, Academic Press, 1971
6. Tom Cox, *Stress.* Baltimore: University Park Press, 1978.
7. Kobasa, Suzanne et al., *Journal of Occupational Medicine,* 21(1979) 595-8.
8. Lazarus, R.S. *Psychological Stress and the Coping Process,* New York: McGraw-Hill, 1966.
9. Pines, Maya, "Psychology Today, December, 1980,
10. Ibid.

CHAPTER TWO

SYSTEMATIC TREATMENT OF CAUSES OF STRESS

To the best of the author's knowledge, there is not currently available for the related professional and the layman alike any systematic analysis of causes of stress. This lack may be partly due to the diversity and abundance of objects and events which may serve as stressors and conditions which predispose any individual to stress. In this and the subsequent chapters the author proposes to remedy the deficiency.

For this purpose, the author has chosen to organize the numerous causes of stress into three main categories: physiological, psychological, and environmental. Obviously, this and any other categorization is bound to be arbitrary; it is imposed on the data, rather than arising from it. Further, it is overly simplistic. Suffice to say, at this point, that any given experience of stress arises, not from any single cause, but from a constellation of interacting causes.

Moreover, the writer knows from his multidisciplinary knowledge that the human being is an open system, equipped with homeostatic mechanisms, which tend to maintain a relatively stable state within the organism and to return it to a steady state whenever it has been disturbed. As a matter of fact, disturbances of the normal condition may arise from within the body or from outside the body. The stressors, which give rise to these disturbances, create the irritating causes of stress. Emotional disturbances arise from a gathering of more or less subtle and subtle stressors, including a wide range of genetic disorders, congenital conditions, and bodily states, which arise in the normal course of living.

There's one additional categorization of the causes of stress which have been discussed in detail in the literature: the division into primary and secondary causes. A primary source of stress may consist of any stimulus or combination of stimuli which triggers the General Adaptation Syndrome (G.A.S.). A key reason jay is either internal or external. The secondary causes of stress consist of those bodily states and activities which are at once the effects of one or more fundamental causes of stress and, as a result of positive feedback, the cause of additional stress. This implies that certain bodily states and conditions, which constitute the effects of one or more basic causes of stress, may in themselves, provide constructive feedback to expand or worsen the demanding conditions. Obviously, the secondary causes of stress are purely psychological.

Some stressors by their exact nature tend to produce effects which in turn, constitute the secondary causes of stress; and some individuals appear to be particularly vulnerable to such primary causes and also prone to produce the real affects which constitute the secondary causes or stress.

Hans Selye referred to these secondary causes of stress as "diseases adaptations". These may take one of two forms: lesions in the organs involved in the "General Adaptation Syndrome", or abnormal responses to such organs. As stated earlier, every stress response has both beneficial and adverse effects. The secondary causes of stress constitute the main source of adverse effects. Any given stress disorder arises not merely from any one or more of the range of possible stressors occurring within the body or environment. Nevertheless, some type of classification of the causes of stress is ideal for bringing some measure of discipline to an otherwise chaotic range of information as a reason for my discussion and for use as a diagnostic tool in understanding the process of stress.

Physiological Theories of Stress

The author has selected for analysis ten categories of the physiological causes of stress, rather than try to deal with specific stressors, which would involve in an effort to produce a continuous enumeration. Though this categorization is not exhaustive, it will be helpful in ordering and presenting the available information on the subject. The author has selected these particular categories because they are the ones most prominently and often mentioned in the literature on stress because they appear, also from the literature, to be the categories of most importance in stress affecting all the profession and the general. The stressors comprised in this category include genetic and hereditary factors; life experience, biological rhythms; sleep; diet; posture; fatigue; muscular tension; disease, and diseases integration.

a. Genetic and Congenital Factors:

Physiological factors, which begin prior to birth, could influence the individual to prone to stress or be causes of stress. The individual's genetic composition is one of these prenatal factors. The susceptibility to hypertension, for example, and a variety of other diseases may be inherited traits. Research has indicated that all of the individual's physical and psychological characteristics, including all of his strengths and/or weaknesses, are controlled to some extent by instructions contained in the body's genetic code. Despite the fact that some individual traits are influenced by environmental factors, the genetic composition constitutes a significant factor in predisposing the individual to certain types of stress

The process of rectal development during pregnancy is a second factor that predisposes the individual to stress. For instance, if the child-bearing mother ingests certain medications, drugs, poisons, alcoholic beverages, and allergenic foods, congenital defects may develop in the baby. Certain diseases such as rubella may also provide such effects. In fact, any internal or external stressor, which the expectant-mother experiences may affect the unborn child adversely, and the result may last the lifetime of the child. The effects may take the form of a variety of tissue weaknesses, organ dysfunction, and abnormal behavior of various kinds.

We can see how one's entire life experience, both the genetic structure and pathological conditions affect all of the other factors that I would be discussing.

b. Biological Rhythms:

There is a significant amount of research being undertaken and reported in the field of biological rhythms. According to Luce (1971) the term "biological rhythms" applies to a subject of scientific research; and must be distinguished from a similar term, biorhythms which if effectively applied to a popular fad without scientific foundations. The basis of biological rhythms research is that the process of change is neither irregular nor chaotic but rhythmic in nature. All types of forces permeate the universe. Examples of such forces are gravitational, electromagnetic and physical. Each of these forces has a steady character of its own. It is necessary to note that all forms of organic matter, including human, conforms to such rhythms and enhance biological rhythms of their own, Luce (1971) argues.

The rhythmic processes range from cycles of a few milliseconds, for cells to much longer for the body as a whole. Most forms of life, including human beings, exhibit circadian rhythms. Over one hundred internal functions of the human body, ranging from pulse rate to temperature to mood and physical and mental capabilities have been identified as operating in a rhythmic mode. These biological rhythms are intricately interrelated and synchronized to ensure a proper state of homeostasis. Luce contends that when the body is subjected to stress these biological rhythms may become uncoupled, thus disturbing the normal balance. The disturbance of the normal balance serves as positive feedback to provide secondary symptoms of stress. Both the primary disturbance and the positive feedback affect the sleep patterns of the individual. In addition, through the life experience, any disturbance in the biological rhythms is likely to have some effect on other factors that would be discusses in this chapter.

c. Life Experience:

According to Levinson (1978) life experience is a process of transitions; some of these transitions present crises for the individual and these are, to some extent always stressful. Each person has his or her own unique life histories, one's own unique set of events, which can be conveniently referred to as one's "life experiences". For example, during childhood we suffer the ravages of the usual childhood diseases, such as measles, or scarlet fever; plus a multitude of accidents which may contain broken bones, and a myriad of other conditions, which range from, pinworms to heart murmurs. In adolescence, children have the problems of adjusting to a developing sense of independence and the phenomena of sex. Levinson (1978) argues that some of the physical changes that occur during this period may lead to emotional stress. People live in a world of constant change, and one is constantly involved in effecting changes, in the universe, but one's mind and body are no exceptions to the law.

Some researchers have suggested that certain types of changes occur at certain stages of life and that such changes constitute crisis. One's life experiences influence how one deals with such crisis.

d. Sleep:

Luce (1971) proposes that sleep is part of the human being's biological rhythm system and is in turn affected by other biological rhythms. If sleep is interfered with it can throw the whole biological process of rhythms out of order. This in turn can worsen the stressful conditions. Moreover, irregular or abnormal sleeping patterns predispose the individual to fatigue, muscle tension, poor posture, various diseases, and some disease adaptations.

e. Diet:

By the term diet, the author implies foods, food supplements, and vitamin preparations ingested by the person for nutritional purposes. Although nutrition is far from being an exact science, there are certain basic facts which have been established and certain basic principles which have been demonstrated to be essential to human health. It is known that a normal person requires a well-balanced diet, including specific proportions of proteins carbohydrates, fats, and vitamins, certain essential minerals and water. The proportions may vary from person to another individual depending on body weight, degree of activity, physical condition, etc, but some amount of the identical nutrients must be included in every diet. Any significant departure from these basic requirements, any critical quantitative or qualitative nutritional deficiency may produce a physical form which acts as a stressor. Overeating, may serve as a cause of stress.

According to Cannon (1963), during the "General Adaptation Syndrome" (G.A.S.) there are significant changes in the blood sugar level, with the body calling strongly in its glucose reserves. Hence, any pre-excision metabolic disorders or deficiencies would tend to exacerbate the effects of stress and vice versa, in a positive feedback cycle.

Selye (1950) maintains that additional dietary deficiencies and overreaction tend to interfere with normal metabolic processes, to disrupt the normal blood sugar levels, and to place undue stress on the homeostatic mechanisms of the body. Such disturbances tend to disturb other biological rhythms and to predispose the individual to fatigue, irregular sleep patterns, and disease. Definite links have been established between certain diseases, and dietary excess of fat, sugar, and salt; too much fat, too much sugar and too much salt, all have been shown to be contributory factors to heart disease, cancer, obesity, and stroke and among, other killing, diseases.

f. Posture:

Posture is the function of the skeletal frame work and the general body musculature, poor posture interferes with the proper functioning of a number of the normal reflexes and may also adversely affect some of the other internal organs and subsystems, such as the cardiovascular system, the respiratory system and the digestive system. It may also adversely affect the individual's emotional well-being, and his or her social intercourse. The erect posture of mankind, which is unique in the animal kingdom, is well suited to locomotion but poorly suited to standing. From this circumstance arise many of the stress stimuli generally suited to poor posture.

Poor posture may be due to one or more of three causes: diseases of the skeletal framework of the body or associated musculature; or improper use of the muscles; or associated musculature; or improper use of the muscles; or disturbances of the vestibular apparatus of the inner ear, through which one regulate one's balance against the force of gravity. Deformities or diseases of bones and muscles may be due to genetic or congenital defects or to eventually acquired injuries or diseases. Whatever the case, the resulting condition may constitute a source of stress by placing excessive demands on certain parts of the body, thereby disturbing the normal homeostasis.

Frequently posture is simply a reflection or expression of certain emotional attitudes; thus good posture is indicative of self-confidence or extroversion, poor posture of lack of confidence and introversion. Disturbances by injury or disease of the vestibular apparatus of the inner ear may result in one's inability to sit, stand, or walk without assistance. Poor posture whatever the cause, tends to stimulate muscular tension and to predispose the individual to fatigue, irregular sleep patterns, and certain diseases, it may also interfere with other biological rhythms.

g. Fatigue:

Technically, fatigue is the name applied to a condition in a sensory receptor or motor end organ characterized by brief loss of power to respond because of repeated or continued stimulation. More generally, it connotes weariness from physical over exertion or nervous exhaustion. At a lower level of analysis, fatigue is characterized by either or both, excessive accumulation of waste products (e.g. Lactic acid) or inadequate supplies of blood sugar and oxygen to the affected part.

The condition may result from a variety of causes, in addition to basic overexertion, for example, excessive smoking or drinking, heart disease, or tuberculosis, any of which may cause fatigue upon mild exertion. Prolonged fatigue may lead to sleep disturbances, muscular tension, poor posture, improper diet, and other forms of lesser stress. It may dispose the body to a number of diseases and interfere with the biological rhythms.

h. Muscular Tension:

There is a close relationship between muscular tension and nervous tension. In fact, the two terms are simply different names for two different aspects of the same psycho physiological phenomenon. Muscular tension is simply a prolonged contraction of the muscles in response to certain emotions (nervous adjustments to life experience) or to postural defects or other chronic conditions. Contraction of the muscles automatically shortens the connective tissue (fascia). Permanent facial shortening or thickening result from habitual muscular tension; tearing of the fascia results from unexpected or improper stretching of the muscles. Both result in pain and other minor stresses.

    A significant source of muscle tension resulting from emotional disturbances is the wide range of petty annoyances and irritations each of us experience every day-loud talk, raucous laughter, having someone cough or sneeze in your face, missing the bus when one is in a hurry, etc. Certain muscles become tense each time we experience such a petty annoyance or intuition. The muscles remain tense and fail to relax as they should in the normal pattern of tensing and relaxing, they lose

i. Muscular Tension:

There is a direct relationship between muscular tension and nervous tension. In fact, the two terms are simply different names for two different aspects of the same psycho physiological phenomenon. Muscular tension is simply a prolonged contraction of the muscles in response to certain emotions (nervous adjustments to life experience) or to postural defects or other pathological conditions. Contraction of the muscles automatically shortens the connective tissue (fascia). Permanent facial shortening or thickening result from chronic muscular tension; tearing of the fascia results from unexpected or undue stretching of the muscles. Both result in pain and other secondary stresses.

A significant source of muscle tension resulting from emotional disturbances is the wide variety of petty annoyances and irritations each of us face every day-loud talk, raucous laughter, having someone cough or sneeze in your face, missing the bus when one is in a hurry, etc. Certain muscles become tense each time we face such a minor irritation or irritation. The muscles remain tense and fail to relax as they should in the normal cycle of tensing and relaxing, they lose resiliency, they become stiff and inelastic if this petty stresses continue to occur throughout the day. Thus, the muscle loses its capacity to release tension as to become permanently shortened. This may lead to a stiff neck, headaches, back pain, and variety of other complaints.

Conversely, muscles, which are insufficiently exercised, tend to become flabby, shortened, and equally inelastic. The weakened muscles may go into spasm or even tear, when the tensions resulting from petty annoyances and irritations occur.

Emotional habit patterns resulting in muscular tension frequently carry over into sleep, depriving the victim of needed sleep. The resulting in muscular tension often carries over into sleep, depriving the victim of needed sleep. The resulting fatigue stimulates further tension in continuing cycle of positive feedback and secondary stress. Thus, emotional responses to any form of stress tend to become habitual establishing such positive feedback cycles.

j. Disease:

Disease if an impairment or disturbance in the function or structure of the body, or one or more parts thereof due to the failure of the adaptative mechanisms to adequately counteract one or more varieties or stressors. According to Claude Bernard (1865), health is a matter of balance, which in turn depends on a relatively constant composition of the inner medium—the "milieu interior". The organism's ability to resist disease is based on the number of complex balancing actions —the homeostatic process of dynamic stabilization that involves many parts of the body working together co-operatively.

The body is more susceptible to stressors such as infectious microbes, when the homeostatic mechanisms are not operating properly. The body is able to resist or overcome invading microbes, when the homeostatic mechanisms are working properly. Thus, in the current approach disease is not a particular state or condition attributable to a single cause; rather, it is a physical process involving the efforts of the homeostatic mechanism to deal with disturbances caused by one or more stressors. The particular physical response depends on a number of factors, including the genetic composition of the individual, previous experience state, etc. In some instances, these responses (the G.A.S) are abnormal and then constitute diseases in themselves. Any disease interferes with normal biological rhythms and tends to induce fatigue, which leads to irregular sleep patterns, muscular tension, and other disturbances.

k. The Adaptation Process:

One of the distinguishing characteristics or organism systems is the capacity for adaptation. Adaptation consists in self-modification to meet the requirements for continued existence under the prevailing conditions of the environment. One of the essential features of the adaptive process is the restriction of the stress response to the minimum amount and area of the body required for maintaining homeostasis. According to Hans Selye (1956), any failure in this process of coping with a stressor results in one or more of the diseases of adaptation.

Any abnormality of the adaptation process itself—any maladaptation—constitutes a disease of adaptation.

The abnormality may take any one of the three forms: inadequate adaptive response (hyper adaptation); excessive adaptive response (hyper adaptation); or, inappropriate response. Inadequate adaptive response may take the form of inadequate secretion of the anti-inflammatory hormones, resulting in such conditions as rheumatic and rheumatoid diseases, certain inflammatory diseases of the skin and eyes, and arthritis. Excessive adaptive response may take the form of overproduction of cortisone hormones, leading to such conditions as cardiovascular disease, and kidney disease. Inappropriate adaptive response consists of any unusual or extraordinary response to stress and may lead to such conditions as nervous and mental diseases, metabolic diseases, cancer or shock. In fact, many common human maladies are diseases of adaptation, consisting of abnormal adaptive responses to stress by one or more organs or subsystems of the body. The disease of adaptation are a form of secondary stress, and as such interfere with the body's ability to provide a normal response to future stressors, thus predisposing the body to the stress involved in all of the factors discussed earlier.

Psychological Theories of Stress

In this section, the author utilize the modeling process, this time as a basis for making clear the systematic nature of the psychological theories of stress, in fact, the most common and the most significant stressors for human beings. This section is, thus, doubly relevant to author's principal argument. Secondly, the model the author present here serves as a basis for his treatment of management of stress in Chapter Four. However, the development of a model of the psychological theories of stress poses particular difficulties.

In the first place, the science of psychology is relatively undeveloped compared to the physical sciences and biology. As a result, the concepts and theories are more fluid, less accepted.

For instance, there continue to be fundamental disagreement on such basic matters as the relationship of mind and brain, with neurosurgeons as well as psychologists taking opposing views on the subject. Some insist on the physical identify of the two. Penfield (1975) and Aaron (1975) are unsure or unwilling to take a stand away from more definitive research findings. There are equally fundamental disagreements about the nature of consciousness and the validity of the concepts of altered states of consciousness, according to Tart (1976). This controversy has a direct bearing on some of the coping mechanisms, such as relaxation and intervention techniques) to be discussed in this book.

Secondly, there are still a number of schools of thought or varieties of approaches to the study of behavior, such as, behaviorism, Gestalt psychology, psychoanalysis, and the controversial new discipline of sociobiology. Such a situation tends to condition both experiments and the interpretation of their results, leading to some degree of uncertainty and controversy.

Furthermore, researchers are seriously hampered by the fact that scientific analysis of the internal operations of the human mind and brain depend, in the end, on the analytical ability of that same device, the human mind and brain. This involves fundamental differences of perspective and level of analysis; we cannot rise to view the operation of mind and brain from a higher level. We cannot gain the perspective which presumably would be available from a metal level of existence. While we can probe and test the brain of another person with electrodes and surgery, we cannot monitor the internal operations of this "black box", only the inputs and outputs. The only brain we know from the inside in one's own and, so far, we have not found any way to establish an objective view of its operations.

In spite of these difficulties, we must in systems analysis of the psychological theories of stress, be concerned with such matters as mind, brain, consciousness, and emotional as well as physical behavior, rational as well as irrational behavior, normal as well as abnormal behavior, conscious as well as unconscious and subconscious behavior; covert as well as overt behavior, that is internal processes and operations of the central nervous system and other bodily systems as well as publicly observable behavior. This model of psychological theories of stress will be constructed on the basis of a concept of the self-system. The system in this model is a highly abstracted representation of the individual component of psychological study: the human organism.

The Self-System Model: There is a need to set forth certain assumptions concerning the operation of the sympathetic nervous system are inherently cybernetic in its mode of operation: that is, a part of the output of the nervous system flows back to serve as input, thus providing a measure of self-control. An additional assumption is that the self-system has inherent powers of self-reorganization. Before further discussion, I assume that the human organism, and the self-model system, operates generally in the manner of the cybernetic model proposed by Powers (1973) in his highly innovative approach to the psychological functioning of the human body.

Powers (1973) proposes the novel thesis that the nervous system is constructed hierarchically so that each level (except the lowest) provides a measure of control which specifies the behavior of lower levels and thus controls its own input. The inputs as modified by the controls constitute one's perceptions—the only "reality" we can understand. The lowest level of hierarchy receives information in the form of sensory stimuli, whose sole characteristic is the intensity; that is all stimuli, internal or external, are distinguishable at the lowest level of the nervous system in terms of intensity only. All other distinctions—quantitative—are made at higher levels in the neurological hierarchy and are conditioned by internal states and processes of the nervous system at those levels.

Within the neurological system, there are continually flowing reference signals, which are constantly, being modified in a cybernetic manner. Each level, except the lowest, provides the reference signals for the next lower level and is dependent on that lower level for its input. In many instances, two or more level provides reference signals for a single lower. If these reference signals are compatible they will serve to reinforce each other, thus providing a stronger input to the lower order level. If these reference signals are in conflict, they will tend to offset each other. When the conflicting signals are equal in strength, they effectively eliminate control within the range defined by their reference levels, thus resulting in a strong avoidance of either reference level.

Each level, including the lowest, provides input to the next higher level. Each level compares its input from the lowest level and reference signal constitutes an error which serves to increase the tension in some particular muscle or muscle group. This change in tension stimulates effort to reduce or correct the error, thus restoring the normal level of control—the homeostatic function suggested by Cannon (1963). The whole process is cybernetic in nature so that both the output and the input signals serve to alter the continually flowing signals.

Anxiety, Arousal, and the Self-Concept: According to Epstein (1973), the individual has a conceptual self-system that, in effect, is an implicit theory that the person has unwittingly constructed about himself. Implicit self-theories are developed as contractual tools for accomplishing certain ends. The basic functions of all self-theories are to maintain a favorable pleasure/pain balance over the foreseeable future to assimilate the data of significant experience, and to keep self-esteem. To the extent that an implicit self-theory to fulfill its functions, the theory is stable, and the person has a sense of well-being and is motivated to the extent of his range of experience. To the extent that an implicit self-theory is unable to fulfill its functions, stress is placed on the organization of the theory. This stress is experienced subjectively as unpleasant arousal, or anxiety, and there is a tendency for disorganization to happen. The threat is reacted to either with one's defenses to reduce the self-theory or by changes in the self-theory that allow it to fulfill its functions more effectively through assimilation of new elements, or change in, or rearrangement of, old elements. If the defense of the self-theory or peripheral changes in it is unsuccessful, stress on the self-theory may escalate until total disorganization occurs. Disorganization can be adaptive because it provides an opportunity for re-organization.

Epstein (1973) argues that the basic postulates in a person's self-theory can be inferred from the nature of his emotions and the events that elicit them. A study of emotions thus provides a useful research approach for investigating the nature of self-theories. There are three primary sources of anxiety: threat to life or limb, threats to the assimilative capacity of a person's conceptual system, and threats to self-esteem. The first is common to all higher order animals, the second is almost exclusively human, and the third is exclusively man. Threats to a person's assimilative capacity (i.e.: failures in assimilation) produce unpleasant arousal, or anxiety; assimilation, however, when it occurs produces unpleasant arousal. Thus, there is a built in the source of motivation for people to expand the scope of their self theories and to assimilate new information. The process is balanced by tension produced perceptions that cannot be assimilated.

The anticipation of, the actual inability of, the self-system to accomplish its functions, places the system under stress, which evokes unpleasant arousal or anxiety. As anxiety mounts, it produces a tendency for the self-system to disorganize or self-destruct. This tendency can be viewed as an adaptive mechanism that arose on the course of evolution as an emergency reaction for correcting a poorly organized complex conceptual system. That is given a limited conceptual framework; its disorganization can pave the way for a sudden, drastic reorganization. Such correction can be contrasted with learning through reinforcement, which is suited to the gradual correction of individual elements within the system. The anticipation of total disorganization is extremely disturbing as it portends disorientation and system at all costs. Threats to self-esteem normally do not produce disorganization. Instead, they evoke coping mechanisms that serve to maintain the stability of the self-system.

Rogers (1971) maintains that there are three broad mechanisms that people use to cope with threats to the self-system. These consist of ignoring or avoiding the implications of a threatening event, distorting the perception of interpretation of the event, and modifying the self-system so that it can assimilate the new information. The first two correspond to defense mechanisms, whereas, the last corresponds to personality growth. Facing events that have implications for changing a person's implicit self-theory is anxiety arousing. However, the actual process of assimilation and its aftermath are associated with a state of pleasant arousal.

Epstein (1973) noted that the factors that determine whether a person will assimilate new information and grow as a personality or be defensive are the body's current level of arousal and its affective tone, the stability and flexibility of his implicit self-theory, previous practice and habits in coping with threat, and the rate and amount of stimulation and whether the stimulation is expected. There is only so much aversive arousal that any person can endure before anxiety becomes overwhelming and disorganization sets in, according to Harlow (1953). Accordingly, a person who is already experiencing a high level of unpleasant arousal will find almost all additional stimulation aversive and will defend himself against such stimulation. Correspondingly, an individual in a pleasant state of arousal well tend to seek out and assimilate new experiences. An individual in a moderate state of unpleasant arousal, depending on other factors, can either be defensive or can react to his state of anxiety as an incentive to re-examine his self-theory. Lindell (1964) stated that there are two factors that must be considered in assessing a person's background level of arousal. One is his relatively enduring state of arousal; the other is the current background of external stimulation or the degree with which a particular threatening event is experienced. There is considerable evidence that the pleasant effect tends to cancel out the negative effect.

Epstein (1973) discusses the characteristics of a robust-theory, one that is able to assimilate new data with minimal defensiveness. Such a self-theory was assumed to rate high on the attributes of a good theory. Of particular importance is the existence of fundamental, or extremely general, postulates that are securely anchored in a network of significant previous experience, so that they are not invalidated. A postulate equivalent to "I am an honest, competent person" is one such postulate. Such basic postulates imbue the self-theory with stability and flexibility at the same time. These must be supplemented by less general postulates that add specificity and directedness to the system and that can be invalidated without serious consequences to the organization of the system. People who lack stable basic postulates in appropriate, combination with expendable minor postulates have either rigid self-systems or ones that are lacking in sufficient framework to guide behavior with any consistency.

Providing all other factors are held constant, some people are more apt to accept the implications of threatening stimuli than others because of direct training and development of a value system which regards facing challenges from within and without as desirable.

Environmental Theories of stress

The environmental causes of stress include all those objects or events which trigger, or contribute to, the stress response in the individual, but which originate outside of the individual. Such objects and events constitute noxious stimuli, but do not necessarily have to penetrate the self-system to initiate the stress response. A person's ambient environment may be divided into three categories: physical, biotic and social.

Among the obvious physical stressors are those which cause wounds, bruises, or other lesions-objects which cause injury when they strike or penetrate the borders of the self-system, including knives, bullets, rocks and other solid objects. Such objects may be directed at us purposely by an aggressor, or may strike us accidentally; the results are the same in terms of stress. Stress has many definitions; some emphasize the stimulus input, and others emphasize the state of the organism. Peptone (1967) argues that the stimulus is considered as the stressor and the state of the organism as stress. Essentially, stress represents some disturbance in the organism which is characterized by physiological changes.

Duffy (1962) and many other investigators have focused attention on a mechanism that may underlie stress reactions characterized by autonomic excitability and changes in heart rate and galvanic skin response (GSR). Such changes are embodied by the concept of arousal. However, Glass and Singer (1972) suggests that adaptation may occur after an initial alarm period, of there may be a gradual shift to a new and high level of physiological input.

The physical environment may have its impact as a stressor either directly or indirectly. Weybrew (1967), classified primary or direct stressors as those "that involve environmental impositions, trauma, or insult which directly strain or stress the adaptive capacities of the neurophysiological system." Excessive noise and temperature are examples of primary stressors. A study by Davis et al (1955) had provided evidence that such primary stressors generate physiological changes. The results revealed complex effects that are not always clear cut in implications for understanding physiological conceptual issues. Heat (e.g. Weybrew, 2967) and noise (Davis, et al., 1955), (Glass & Singer, 1972), however, appear to induce an autonomic excitability effect. Blood pressure, heart rate, muscle tension and palm sweating increase following the initial reception of excessive noise or heat. Cold results primarily in a reverse pattern of effects, effects, although some responses such as heart rate are congruent with those of heat.

Secondary or indirect stressors are "those environmental circumstances that impose immediate or anticipated barriers to ongoing goal activity" (Weybrew, 1967). These would include violations of personal space (density or proximity), as well as goal blocking. In view of the direct nature of their influence, and the complexity of additional factors they might engage, specification of the effects of secondary stressors may be more complicated than in the case of primary stressors. For example, density produced inconsistent physiological changes in both animal and human.

Freedman (1973) reviewed numerous animal experiments suggesting only some consistent physiological changes, namely endocrine changes. Similarly, results from studies of proximity in dyad and density, in groups, (Dabbs, 1971; Epstein and Aiello, 1974) yielded divergent conclusions. Heshka et al. (1975) attempted to reconcile the conflicting results by showing that the nature of the social situation affected tractions to density.

As predicted, they found that when a peer gazed at the subject in a hostile way, the subject's arousal increased as the peer's proximity increased, whereas when a peer gazed at a subject in a friendly way, the subject's arousal decreased as the peer's proximity increased. It is evident that further exploration of the social context that interacts with density to enhance arousal is needed, particularly in relation to concomitant behavioral changes. Effects can be offset of cognitive factors. Joy et al., (1962) observed that psycho-physiological responses to close were altered by the subject's interpretation of a cold environment or his attitudes toward the experiment. Furthermore, Glass and Singer (1972) reported that GSR adaptation was faster in response to predictable compared with unpredictable noise. Thus, it appears that cognitive appraisal (Lazarus, 1967) about the environmental factor significantly arrests whether it produces a stress reaction.

The Social Environment and Stress

By far the most prolific source of stress to humans is humans themselves—humans in organized society. In my earlier listing of the physical stressors, I have included a number which are direct or indirect consequences of social and urban living. Other consequences of the modern life style also constitute stressors. Both the scientific and the popular literature are replete with reports of the stressful effects of the workplace (monotony, production pressure, inept bosses, etc. of the leisure world (insufficient time for some individuals, ineffective use of leisure time by others, overexertion in some activities, overly aggressive pursuit of some avocations, etc.), and of the natural environment (devastation, pollution, etc.).

The crowded conditions of some of the cities lead to stress; there is a source of stress in simple over-population. The very pace of urban living leads to stress and that pace appear to be accelerating. The increasing frequency in changes in jobs, occupations, employer, placed of residence, all lead to lack of personal stability, to lack of stable relationships, and to stress. The rate of innovation and the sheer volume of innovation lead to stress—to what Toffler (1970) calls "future shock".

For the professional, the problems involved in the management of change constitute a source of stress; any break with tradition, any discontinuity, serves as a source of stress for employees. The management of time by the teacher or the nurse, including his or her leisure time, is a source of stress.

Certain individuals, groups, organizations and intuitions are more significant than others as sources of stress for the teacher or the nurse—those who interact with him or her continually or frequently. This category of "significant others" includes bosses, family members, colleagues, professional associates, friends, acquaintances, neighbors; as well as informal groups (of friends, associates, etc.) and formal groups (employing organizations, religious and fraternal organizations, civic organizations, etc.). It also includes other groups and organizations of which the professional (i.e. the nurse or the teacher) is not a member, but which he or she interacts as customer, rival, client, patron, citizen, etc.

Glass and Dinger (1972) argue that the bureaucratic milieu (school or hospital) is in itself stressful whether one is working in it or dealing with it from the outside. Established social institutions (rules, laws, folkways, mores, etc.) impose restrictions on the individual and limit freedom of action in a wide variety of ways, many of which may be perceived as stressful. Rules and customs of etiquette or protocol are simply prescription for conduct, which if not followed constitute the source of stress for the individual.

Another reason for the stressful effects is the fact that within the accepted body of principles one may find numerous inconsistencies, pairs of principles which are mutually contradictory. Some principles, for example, advocate punitive measures to secure compliance or conformity, while others favor a more humanistic approach. Thus, the teacher or the nurse (and many other professionals) may find himself or herself caught between conflicting guidelines; the resulting uncertainty may leas to immobility and the consequent stressful effects that would be discussed in detail, in chapter three. The professional teacher or the nurse, who blindly try to follow these principles, without giving sufficient though to the consequences, may find themselves in even deeper trouble when they discover that the principles do not apply to the given situation or that they have misapplied them. The results may be equally stressful.

Schon (1967) said that the self-system interacts with the ambient environment in many other ways; in fact, in an infinite variety of ways, including all the ways mankind has devised for working, loafing, eating, and sleeping. For the teacher or the nurse (and for other professionals), work probably provides the most opportunities for interaction and may well be the greatest source of environmental stress. Although most individuals exercise a considerable degree of control over the activities in which they engage, the note-worthy activity of exception is the work, where the individual's behavior may be programmed to a far greater extent than many are willing to admit.

Summary

An analysis of the theories of the physiological, psychological and environmental causes of stress all suggest that any event –within the self-system or in the ambient environment –and even the sheer process of change itself may operate as a stressor on the self-system. Rarely, if ever, however, is there a single stressor triggering the General Arousal Syndrome (G.A.S.) More typically, a combination of stressors operate to trigger the reaction.

Not only do stressors act in concert to trigger the G.A.S., but, as have not been noted earlier, there is often a cascading of effects, with one stressful physiological, or psychological condition leading to another; for example, poor posture leading to fatigue, muscle tension, sleeplessness, etc. Improper diet; jealousy leading to anger or rage, worry and anxiety; loss or bereavement leading to worry, fear and anxiety may all lead to diseases of adaptation. Likewise, some of the physiological conditions lead to psychological effects and vice versa; environmental causes lead to both physiological and psychological effects.

In each instance, of course, the underlying basic stress reaction is the same, the G.A.S. Only the mediate effects are different, for different individuals, and for the same individual at different times. The reasons for these differences, as discussed previously, are several. First, because of the constraints of time and space and the inherent nature of the perceptual process, no two individuals can ever experience precisely the same micro level event. Secondly because of individual differences in the content of the memory store and the internal operation of the self-system (the nature of the internally flowing neural reference signals) no two individuals will ever experience precisely the same perception of any two or more similar events. Thirdly, because the individual and his memory store are continuously changing with new experience, no person will ever have precisely the same perceptions or experiences.

Thus, whether any given event (or series of events) operates as a stressor depends, not only in the nature of that particular event (or series of events) but on two other factors, as well. One of those factors is the vulnerability of the individual to that particular event at the time of its impact (perceived or non-perceived). The other factor is the context that is the individual's perception of the ambient environment in which the event occurs.

According to McLean (1975), stress occurs when there is sufficient overlap among the three factors in a stress situation, namely, stressors, vulnerability and context. The body's vulnerability to a particular stressor depends, on the state of his or her self-system, his age, genetic and cultural development, occupation, education, memory store, physical condition, physical condition, psychological mood, etc. The context of a particular potential traumatic event depends on the nature of the potential stressor itself and the perspective of the individual. Within the family, the workplace, or any other organization, the context of a potential stressor depends on the particular perspective of the individual. The individual is a unique product of genetic, physical, psychological, and cultural development; therefore, vulnerabilities and context will vary from individual to individual, and from moment to moment. This unique quality of each stressful event may provide us with a lead to developing the means of controlling, or managing, stress, which would be the subject of detail discussion later in this book The next chapter will deal with the manifestations and effects of stress.

References

1. Selye, Hens. *Stress without Distress.* Philadelphia, Lippincott, 1974.
2. Luce, Gay Gear. *Body Time: Physiological Rhythms and Social Stress.* New York: Random House, 1971.
3. Luce, Gay G. *Biological Rhythms in Human and Animal Physiology.* New York: Dover, 1971.
4. Levinson, Daniel. *The Seasons of a Man's Life.* New York: Knoff, 1978.
5. Luce, Gay G. *Biological Pythons in Human and Animal Physiology.* New York: Dover, 1971.
6. Berger, Louis, et al. *The Effects of Stress on Dreams.* New York: International Universities, 1971.
7. Cannon, Walter. *The Wisdom of the Body.* Rev. Ed. New York: Norton Library paperback, 1963.
8. Selye, Hans. *Stress.* Montreal: ACTA Medical Publishers, 1950.
9. Novey, Theodore B. *Making Life Work: Transactional Analysis and Management.* Sacramento, Calif.: VAKMAR, 1973.
10. Selye, Hans. *The Stress of Life.* New York: McGraw-Hill Book Co., 1956.

11. Carr, Rachel. *The Yoga Way to Release Tension.* New York: Coward, McCann and Geoghegan, 1974.
12. Bernard, Claude (1865). *An Introduction to the Study of Experimental Medicine.* Henry Copley Greene, Trans. New York: Dover, 1957 (reprint).
13. Cox, Tom. *Stress.* Baltimore: University Park Press, 1980.
14. Penfield, Wilder. *The Mystery of the Mind.* Princeton, N.Y: Princeton University, 1975.
15. Tart, Charles. *State of Consciousness.* New York: Dutton, 1975.
16. Powers, William T. *Behavior: The Control of Perception.* Chicago, Ill.: Aldine, 1973.
17. Epstein, S. "Toward a unified theory of anxiety" in B. Maher (ed.) *Progress in Experimental Personality Research.* Vol.4. New York: Academic Press,
18. Epstein, S. "The self-concept revisited, or a theory of a theory". *The American Psychologist.* 1973, Vol.28.
19. Rogers, C. R. *Client-centered Therapy.* New York: Houghton Mifflin, 1951.
20. Harlow, H. F. & Zimmerman, R.R. "Affectionate responses in the infant monkey". *Science.* 1959, Vol. 130,
21. Lindell, H.S. "The role of vigilance in the development of animal neurosis." In P.H. Hock & Zubin (Eds). *Anxiety.* New York: Hafner, 1964.
22. Pepitone, A.: Self, social environment and stress". In M.H. Appley & R. Trumbull (Eds). *Psychological Stress* New York: Appleton-Century-Crofts, 1967.
23. Glass, D.C. and Singer, J. R. *Urban Stress.* New York: Academic Press, 1972.
24. Davis, R.C., et al. "Automatic and muscular responses and their relation to simple stimuli". *Psychological Monographs,* 1955. 65 (20 Whole No. 405).
25. Freedman, J. The effects of population density on human. In J. Fawcett, (ed.) *Psychological Perspectives on Population.* New York: Basic Books, 1973.

26. Heshka, S. et al. A proximity and arousal in social encounters. Paper presented at the meeting of the Canadian Psychological Association, Quebec City, and June 1975.
27. Stokols, D. "On the distinction between density and crowding. Some implications for further research" *Psychological Review,* 1972.
28. Loo. C. "Important issues in researching the effects of crowding on humans." *Representative Research in Social Psychology* 1973, Vol.4.
29. Lazarus, R.S. Cognitive and personality factors underlying threat and coping. In M.H. Appley &R. Trumbull (eds.) *Psychological Stress.* New York: Appleton-Century-Crofts, 1967.
30. Toffler, Alvin. *Future Shock.* New York: Random House, 1970.
31. Schon, Donald A. *Technology and Change.* New York: Delacorte, 1967.

CHAPTER THREE

MANIFESTATIONS AND EFFECTS OF STRESS

Manifestations of Stress

The only way we can recognize the state of any system is by the evidence it provides through one's sensory apparatus, its appearances and manifestations. Thus, the state of stress can only be recognized; by the way, it reveals itself to one's senses, by its manifestations. The process involves in the stress response can be understood by analyzing the system, dissect it and examine (physically and mentally) the separate parts and their interactions. Selye (1950) and a number of other investigators have provided us with verbal and graphic reports so that we need to perform only the mental dissection, reading their reports. What follows is a synthesis of the currently available information.

Perhaps, the most dramatic example of manifestations of stress may be found in an imaginative description of the phenomenon as it might have been experienced by one of one's prehistoric ancestors. If a Mesolithic caveman unexpectedly encountered an aggressive wild animal, such as saber-toothed tiger, his body would immediately activate what today's physiologists commonly refer to as, the "fight or flight response," also variously termed, the "alarm reaction", by Selye (1950) or the "emergency response" by Cannon (1939). The hairs on the caveman's head and body would tend to become erect, his heart would pound harder and faster, his breathing would become deeper, his pupils would dilate, and he would become mentally more alert. The reaction, including all these symptoms, would be almost instantaneous. There are, of course, innumerable other types of threats of a subliminal nature which may just as effectively serve to arouse the stress response, although with somewhat different superficial symptoms; for example, invasion of the body by stressor agents such as harmful viruses or bacteria.

The General Adaptation Syndrome (G.A.S) is a highly complex series of interacting events, which constitute the, human response to any stressor; the following paragraphs summarize the principal findings of Selye and other investigators, omitting the highly technical clinical details. Selye (1950) maintains that G.A.S. consists of three principal stages. The first stage which he termed, the "alarm reaction" is elicited upon sudden exposure to stressors to which the body is not qualitatively or quantitatively adapted. This stage has two distinct sub stages: (1) the shock sub stage, characterized by the "fight of flight reaction" and (2) the counter shock sub stage, characterized by a reversal of the initial fight or flight symptoms, and certain internal organic changes. In the first stage, according to Selye (1950), the general resistance of the body to the particular stressor tends to drop below normal. In the second stage, the self-system begins to adapt to the stressor through a gradual increase in resistance to it and a decrease in resistance to other stimuli. The third stage is that of exhaustion, the self-system is no longer able to maintain the state of adaptation. This third stage may be a precursor to death if stress continues for long enough periods.

Earlier the author has discussed the variety of objects and events which may act as stressors. It was noted earlier that any noxious agent which assaults the self-system or even any event which is perceived as a threat to the self-system may serve as a stressor which trigger the alarm reaction. The response is essentially the same regardless of whether the stimulus involves physical assault or only a perception (optical, auditory, olfactory, or other) involving the release of a complex series of neural and hormonal messages, which in turn activate a number of glands, organs and other subsystems of the body.

There is no complete information about the exact nature or chemical composition of the alarm signals, although there is no doubt about their occurrence. The last word is not in on the neural or chemical nature of the messages going to the hypothalamus and the pituitary gland, the central control organs of the G.A.S. It is, however, known that some sort of neural hormonal alarm signals emanate from the site of the directly affected body cells when the stressor strikes, either physically or perceptually.

The alarm signal is neural and flows from the directly affected sensory area if the stressor is perceptual in nature. On the contrary, the immediate reaction takes the form of a local adaptation syndrome (L.A.S.) if the stressor is physical in nature. As a result, some of the cells or tissues of the directly stressed area may die and the surrounding tissues become inflamed. The blood vessels in the affected area are dilated, fluids and bloods leak out from the dilated blood vessels into the surrounding tissues. In response to the irritation from the stressor, the cells of the fibrous connective tissue begin to multiply rapidly. Chemical substances are then secreted by the blood vessels and the connective tissues which tend to offset the irritating effects of the stressor, and which destroy any invading microorganisms. The area then becomes inflamed, reddened and heated as a result of this multiplication of cells and fluids. The nearby nerve ending become irritated by all this activity causing the sensation of pain. The whole process constituted the body's vigorous defense against the stressor, the fight response. It tends to produce a barricade around the stressed area to prevent the spread of the invader.

Meanwhile, one or more alarm signals emanate from the directly stressed area. The neural signals of distress flow to the brain, perhaps, first to the cortex and then to the hypothalamus, perhaps directly to the hypothalamus; then to the pituitary. Certain hormones (noradrenalin and acetylcholine (ACH) are released by the nerve endings. These hormones act locally but may also carry distress signals directly to other organs and subsystems.

Lying at the junction of the midbrain and the thalamus is a very small but vitally organ called the hypothalamus. The hypothalamus is, perhaps, the most prominent structure involved in the control of the autonomic nervous system; it plays a vital role on the experiencing of emotions and motivations. It contains a number of critical regulatory centers, and it is mainly responsible for controlling body temperature. The hypothalamus activates the adrenal medulla, the autonomic nervous system, and through the pituitary gland, the endocrine system, when appropriately stimulated by an alarm signal.

Upon activation by the hypothalamus, the pituitary gland secretes several hormones, three of which are crucial in the G.A.S. One of these hormones—adrenocorticotropin (ACTH)—activates the adrenal cortex. Another hormone called throtropin (TTH) activates the thyroid gland. The third hormone known as vasopressin (ADH) tends to increase the blood pressure by acting on unstirred muscles of, and thereby constricting the blood vessels.

The adrenals are two bean-shaped glands located one above each kidney; they are endocrine (ductless) glands. When stimulated by ACTH, the adrenal cortex secretes two other types of hormones, ones (anti-inflammatory corticoids; and pro-inflammatory corticoids. It is known that the pro-inflammatory corticoids promote inflammation and influence mineral metabolism. The anti-inflammatory corticoids inhibit inflammation and increase the blood sugar level. While these hormones sometimes oppose each other, as in their impact on inflammation, at other times they may act synergistically. For example, they may have a detrimental effect on the kidneys, producing inflammation, and renal lesions, which in turn cause a significant increase in blood pressure. Their specific activities depend, in each instance, on the nature of the threat and the nature and extent of activity of other organs and glands.

By raising energy levels in the stress response by accelerating chemical reactions throughout the body, the thyroid gland directly controls the metabolism rate. The hormone thyroxin is secreted by the thyroid; thyroxin makes body tissues more sensitive to adrenaline (epinephrine) a hormone secreted by the adrenal medulla.

The autonomic nervous systems: Noradrenalin (nor epinephrine) is secreted or released at the sympathetic nerve termination. Noradrenalin tends to inhibit the activity of the smooth muscles of the alimentary canal; accelerates the heart beat; dilate the bronchi, so that oxygen is drawn into the lungs; and it dilates, the pupils of the eye so that more light is allowed in. These nerve fibers will also serve to dilate some blood vessels and constrict others. Acetylcholine (ACH) is secreted by the parasympathetic nervous system, which tend to counteract the effects of noradrenalin (nor epinephrine), thus, serving to restore normal functioning when the crisis has passed the homeostatic effect.

Adrenaline (epinephrine) is secreted when the inner core of the adrenals is stimulated. Adrenaline tends to stimulate the heart, constrict the blood vessels, and delay muscle fatigue. Adrenaline is identical with noradrenalin, a hormone secreted at the sympathetic nerve ending), but while the latter has a purely local significance, the adrenaline secreted by the adrenal medulla has an overall effect on the self-system since it is secreted into the blood stream and circulates through the body.

All this activity places the body in a heightened state of alertness, with an increased blood supply, glucose, and oxygen to the brain muscles, and other organs and tissues, and increased efficiency of the perceptual apparatus. Thus, the body is ready to fight or flee as additional events may dictate.

The fact that this sequence of events is non-specifically produced is of particular significance. To a greater or lesser degree, it occurs whenever the self-system is sufficiently disturbed or is required to respond to unexpected demands. The stressor agent may be as evidently innocuous as strenuous exertion of the muscles, in work or recreational activities; or may be in the kind of mental or emotional demands associated with a new job or traumatic event; or an invasion of the body by a noxious agent; or any other event which requires a significant adjustment of the internal operations of the self-system.

Inflammation may occur following any injury, perceived threat, or activity of the body or one or more of its subsystems, which is more, widespread than normal, with resulting stiffness and pain. The characteristic response is a key feature of the self-system's ability to adapt to changes in its ambient conditions or to local demands. The self-system tends to restrict the traumatic effects to the smaller area of the body consistent with meeting the requirements for restoring homeostasis. For example, inflammation serves to limit an attacker to the immediate area of attack, and to remove the resulting debris. The more extensive area of arrack and the greater the amount of tissue damage, the greater is the self-system responded (in the production of adrenocortitropine and other hormones).

Subsystems

The subsystems, hormones, organs and glands, mentioned earlier perform other functions. They interact in a variety of ways to create a synergistic effect during the stress response. This suggests that any other proposed set of the self-system into subsystems for descriptive purposes is arbitrary and depends on the perspective of the observer.

A number of glands, organs, and other parts of the body perform various functions and some functions are performed by a number of parts acting alone or in concert. Furthermore, a significant aspect of Selye's (1950) opinion, the General Adaptation Syndrome (G.A.S.) involves not just parts of the body I have discussed elsewhere in this chapter, but every other part of the body in one way or another, directly or indirectly. Of course, this becomes apparent when we realize that both the composition and the rate of flow of the blood (which carries a number of hormones and other substances) and the level of activity of the entire nervous system are involved on the G.A.S. and that every cell and organ in the body depend on these two integrators of physical activities.

In addition to participating in controlling the glucose level of the blood, the liver is one of the principal controllers of the degree of concentration of a variety of other chemical substances such as proteins, insulin and certain hormones. It serves as a sort of warehouse, storing reserves of carbohydrates for conversion to glucose as needed; it also destroys excess quantities of the corticoid hormones.

Certain white blood calls (e.g. the lymphoid cells and the eosinophils) participate in the G.A.S. by regulating serologic immune reactions and the level of sensitivity to allergens. Practically every aspect of the self-system so involved in the General Adaptation Syndrome (G.A.S.), although the key elements involved are the nervous system, the pituitary gland, the thyroid gland, the adrenals, the liver, and the kidneys, in addition to the cells of the directly affected tissues.

Joseph Nii Abekar Mensah, PhD.

Multiple Effects

It is difficult, if not difficult to detect and understand all of the various effects of the three stages in the General Adaptation Syndrome throughout the body, in view of the differences in stressors. Some effects are specific, some non-specific; some local, some general; some benign, some malign; however, in a biologic systems complex as the human body such distinctions may not always be clearly identifiable. Any given outcome may be, at once confined in one aspect and general in another. Such effect may be beneficial to specific organs or tissues and harmful to others. Besides, there are both specific and non specific effects and certain specific effects may upset or even stop entirely, individual specific effects in any given instance, any time a stressor acts upon a specific target. When a stressor acts upon different targets, each will produce both specific and nonspecific effects; the latter will be additive because the alarm signals are the same, but the specific effects will not be additive because the individual responses are different.

However, it is not the intent of the author to seek any comprehensive survey of the multiple effects of stress in this book. Certain effects of the General Adaptation syndrome (G.A.S.) are also serious than others for the discussions. At this time, I will clearly identify these more serious effects in a basis for more specific talk later in this study.

Stress response does not always conform to the normal pattern. Certain diseases of adaptation may occur when the stress response deviates significantly, failing to cope adequately with a stressor. Successful adaptation signifies the completion of a new level of homeostasis in consonance with the ambient environment; it involves a properly balanced combination of defending or passive measures by the body or the involved elements thereof. Disease may occur when the body fails to provide such a balance or when there is excessive defensive or passive response. The excessive defensive reaction may appear in the form of hyperactivity or overdevelopment in a certain aspect (e.g. allergic reactions); excessive submission may result from exhaustion or failure of the element to respond (e.g. renal failure). Such extreme responses (defensive or passive) could also be emotional rather than physical in nature, taking the form of worry, anger, depression, etc.

Inappropriate responses, therefore, by the body during the stress response are diseases of adaptation. They are the indirect result of attacks by stressors, in contrast to other diseases resulting from such attacks. Of course, the distinction is largely conceptual since the body rarely, if ever successfully responds to any significant stressors without some degree of maladaptation. This implies that there are no "pure" diseases, in which only the directly affected organ is involved, with no side effects on other organs —no pure heart disease, kidney disease, etc.

Among the most notable result of stress are the cardiovascular changes. The most obvious, immediate aftermath of stress is inflammation, a fundamental feature of all diseases, as well as the local response to pain. Inflammation is a syndrome characterized by a variety of symptoms, including swelling, reddening, heat, pain and general interference with function; it is not indicating a response of the body to attack by blood and other body fluids into the affected area.

As indicated earlier, this local response is accompanied by the secretion of a variety of hormones throughout the body, leading to an increased demand for blood in some places, decreased demands in other places, and significant changes in the chemical composition of the blood. Increased blood pressure, blood flow and capillary permeability also accompany this local reaction. Oxygenation and nutrition of all bodily tissues, including those of the heart and blood vessels they are directly affected by these cardiovascular changes.

Significant inflammatory and other changes in the walls of the blood vessels themselves (conditions know as arteriosclerosis) derive from these increased demands on the cardiovascular system, as well as the effects of the increased flow of pro-inflammatory and anti-inflammatory corticoids in the blood. Numerous and diversified local lesions throughout the body (including the heart and the blood vessels themselves) may result, of such vascular derangements are severe enough to happen often enough.

Similarly, excessive demands for oxygen may lead to congestion, edema (excess fluid), and other disturbances of the lungs, resulting in pneumonia and other disorders of the pulmonary system, which, like other elements is subject to inflammation when overworked. The negative effects ramify through other element of the self-system as the supply of oxygen is gradually reduced because of impaired lung functioning.

All parts of the body, including the entire nervous system, depend upon the blood supply for nutrition and oxygen, and being particularly vulnerable to biochemical changes, which occur throughout the body, during the General Adaptation Syndrome (G.A.S.), is particularly vulnerable to the effects of systemic stress. Inflammation and other significant structural and functional derangement in the stress response, with increased activity in the secretion of noradrenalin an acetylcholine at the nerve endings. In addition to these physiological effects, there are the psychosomatic effects of stress resulting from misunderstanding or improper assessment of the importance of other stress reactions, or from the fear of, or worry over, an inability to understand physical conditions or reactions.

The gastro-intestinal tract is also highly sensitive to the effects of stress. This is due, in large part, to severe neural discharges from the autonomic nervous system during the General Adaptation Syndrome. At the same time, the hormones being released tend to stimulate the production of peptic enzymes thereby increasing the onslaught of the digestive juices on the stomach lining. The results often take the form of bleeding ulcers in the stomach and adjacent areas of the alimentary canal.

Thus, the General Adaptation Syndrome (G.A.S.) involves an almost complete mobilization of the body resources so that the strain of increased demands on the self-system is realized in almost every subsystem of the body. For example, the kidneys are subject to greater demands in disposing of the increased amount of waste products resulting from the high rate of metabolism, and in regulating the heightened blood pressure. The strain of these demands makes the kidneys more susceptible to the damaging effects of the corticoid hormones, resulting in irritation, inflammation and renal lesions. The lesions, in turn, constrict the blood vessels of the kidney causing further damage, including histological changes. This constriction of the blood vessels in the kidneys tend to further increase the secretion of renal presser substances, which in turn increase the blood pressure but more by further restricting the blood vessels, and so on in a positive feedback cycle. The sensory systems of the body are also made more vulnerable to inflammatory, allergic, and other disturbances because of the increase demands of the G.A.S., and the consequent elimination of certain white blood cells (lymphoid and eosinophil) which are necessary for production of immunity and in certain allergic reactions.

Also, muscle tones and fatigability as well as the epidermis, hair and nails (resulting in excessive wrinkling, loss of hair, premature graying, etc.) are adversely affected by the heightened level if tension. Osteoporosis may result from the loss of valuable minerals by the skeletal system. The sex organs may also undergo some diminution of activity. The rheumatoid and rheumatic diseases are also expected to maladaptation, of inappropriate reactions to stress. The anti-inflammatory corticoids also diminish one's defenses against certain, usually innocuous, microbes which inhabit one's lungs, skin, and gastrointestinal system and help the body in disposing of dead cells and tissues.

However, it is vital to note that while the basic patterns of the G.A.S. are always the same; there are significant variations in the degree of response and the after-effects among individuals, and for any one person from time to time. There are also variations, in any one person, in the reactivity of different subsystems, organs, glands and cells, These variations are due to such factors as heredity, diet, the current state of health (generally and of the individual organs), previous exposure to stress in general, the specific kind of stress, and other personal, cultural, and environmental factors.

There is also the possibility that repeated exposure to a given, specific stressor may result in selective conditioning of the individual or of certain of his or her subsystems. Such selective conditioning may be positive or negative, increasing or decreasing susceptibility to the specific stressor, raising or lowering the response threshold, enhancing or reducing one's tolerance of stress in general, and in improving or impairing the rate of recovery from stress. Hence the wide variation in nature and extent of response to specific stressors, in the long effects of continued or repeated exposure to stress, and in the ability to manage one's stress levels. In addition to these individual differences in susceptibility, tolerance, and recovery, there is the factor of the duration of exposure to the stressor. For example, repeated brief exposure may tend to increase the amount of tolerance or resistance while exposures of a longer period may tend to be additive in nature, lowering the resistance and increasing the negative effect. Finally, the individual's sense of coping (or failing to tackle) with stress will significantly alter the effects.

Effects of Stress

Considering the relatively formidable variety of causes and effects of stress, one might be deterred from making any attempt at classification were it, not for one fact; the under lying uniformity of the stress reaction. To reiterate, although the particular manifestations of stress will depend on the variable effects of the specific actions of the stressor, the stability and responsiveness of each intermediate physiological subsystem on the self-system, regardless of what particular stressor sets the G.A.S. mechanism is motion, the basic answer is always essentially the same. But the mediate effects are unknown.

Mediate Effects

My focus will be on the main mediate effects of stress on the individual, name and how he copes with stress.. In view of the complexity of interaction among the various type of causes and consequent cascading effects, any attempt to relate specific categories of causes, or even to direct effects would be pointless. For this reason, the author will limit the categories to those which have been widely recognized in the literature as serious and at least potentially measurable. The principal mediate effects identified in the texts are six in number as described in the following paragraphs. I have already suggested the enormous range of physiological and emotional illnesses produced by excessive stress. These then create the first category of direct effects: illness, physical and mental.

It is quite obvious that some of these illnesses may cause the subjects accident-prone. Indeed, some of the under-ling causes, such as fatigue (mental and physical), sleeplessness, anxiety, fear, etc. clearly indicates predisposes their victims to higher accident rates. The second category is then: accidents. It has already been demonstrated that some of the illnesses may result in suicide or death by other means. Death is the third category.

Almost equally obvious, many of these causes and immediate effects may lead directly to lowered effectiveness and efficiency, which becomes the fourth category. Perhaps less obvious is the ways in which the causes and immediate effects lead to the phenomena of turnover and non-turnover, the last two categories of mediate effects. However, the literature is replete with examples of these effects. These then are the six key mediate effects of stress.

<u>Illness:</u> As noted earlier, there are two basic types of stress-related damage to a self-system: (1) direct mechanical damage to tissues which occur almost regardless of the nature of the stress response; and (2) diseases of adaptation, resulting from improper responses by the self-system to a stressor. Even though, the distinction is largely conceptual; in actual practice it becomes difficult, if not impossible, to relate the various effects to their respective causes. Either type of damage may take one or more of three forms of illness or diseases: (1) physiological, (2) psychological, and (3) psychosomatic. The distinctions are not clear cut in either the medical or popular literature, and I shall make no attempt to resolve the defect. Instead, I would adopt the common practice of simply designating any illness or disease as either physical or mental, bearing in mind that the classification is arbitrary.

<u>Physical Illness</u>. Earlier I identified ten key categories of the physiological causes of stress. I also suggested the potential cascading effects of either a negative or post-active impact of any single disturbance of the normal homeostatic balance of the self-system. Improper posture, fatigue, muscle tension, improper diet, insufficient sleep or other disturbances of normal biological rhythm may predispose a person to a variety of disease and disease adaptation. These conditions, in turn, create disturbances which may lead to other diseases and other diseases of adaptation in a continuing cycle, so that the person becomes more and more susceptible to the adverse effects of stress.

The author does intend to go into clinical detail on this subject, but I should mention some of the widely recognized stress-related conditions which have a relatively high level of prevalence among the professions. Alexander (1950) contends that the literature on stress-related research is replete with evidence of stress-related nature of such disease conditions as: migraine, hypertension, hyperthyroidism, heart disease, arthritis, asthma, colitis, diarrhea, constipation, peptic ulcer, insomnia, and possibly diabetes. Although this listing is not exhaustive, it is enough to reflect the wide ranging adverse physiological effects of stress.

<u>Mental Illness</u>: Some or possibly all, of these physical ailments mentioned above may, in any given instance, be psychosomatic in nature; they may have no discernible organic basis, but may be apparently due to some emotional distress from stress.

Such emotional disturbances may in themselves constitute or may lead to illness or diseases. Of course, some mental illness may also be organic in nature somatogenic disorders. The various mental disorders number in hundreds, most of which have no relevance to this discussion. Stress related metal disorders may include certain personality disorders, and certain psycho-physiologic disorders, none of which may occur without appreciable stress. Freedman, Kaplan, and Shaddock (1972) and many other investigators agree on the fact that stress can lead to mental illness. Flash (1974) argues that depression is one type of mental illness, which often, results from improper stress.

Depression

Depression is a syndrome, and not a particular illness or mental disorder; it is a collection of symptoms characterized by a variety of mental disorders.

The symptoms of depression vary from person to person, and from time to time. Depressive symptoms may include a general lowering of mood, including feelings of painful dejections, sadness, loneliness, or apathy; difficulty in thinking;

and psychomotor retardation, including anorexia, insomnia, and loss of libido. Sometimes, symptoms of depression include worry, anxiety, guilt, and a variety of regressive and self-punitive desires. Occasionally, the general retardation may be disguised by periods of restlessness or agitation. Some or any of these symptoms may occur, to a certain degree, in the normal state. Furthermore, some or all of these symptoms may occur in any form of neurotic or psychotic states, which creates some difficulty in classification.

The duration of the disease is also crucial; it may last for just a few weeks or it may persist for months, sometimes remaining chronic indefinitely with periods of temporary remission. Similarly, the intensity of depression may vary from mild discouragement, through despondence, to utter despair; or it may vary from one level to another. The rapidity of onset may also vary, being either sudden or immediate (e.g. following a specific loss or bereavement, or gradual, building up several weeks or months.)

One of the most significant features of the illness is the frequency with which it leads to attempted suicide. The motivation may differ from a desire for relief from the accompanying anxiety to crave for attention, or the attempt may stem from the victim's sense of utter hopelessness. According to Seligman (1975), one of the underlying reasons for the frequent attempts at suicide by depressed persons may be the distorted image they have of themselves, or their idealistic view of the environment, or their future. Depressed individuals tend to see themselves as unattractive and failures, they are deeply pessimistic about their opportunities for the future; the prospect is one of eternal misery.

<u>Accidents</u>: Any condition (physical or mental), which interferes with, an individual's full and free exercise of his or her normal abilities and faculties will lead him or her to accidents. Thus, certain of the causes of stress (e g. Sleeplessness,

fatigue, poor posture, etc), stress itself and specific effects of stress (various physical and mental illnesses, all may lead to the development of proneness to accidents.

Dudley and Welke (1977) cite numerous studies, which show that, the overly aggressive, the frustrated, the passive, and the over-stresses have more frequent automobile accidents. The stress may even be the result of an actual or imminent happy event (a promotion, a marriage etc.) as well as harmful one. In each of these types, the behavior appears to stem from an underlying anxiety produced by the person's fears or worry about his or her ability to measure up to expectations, to perform adequately, Dudley and Welke argue.

Other studies also involve accident-proneness to stress. The accident-prone individual is in general, emotionally less mature, less responsible, more antisocial, and not so well adjusted as those who are less accident-prone. Anxiety resulting from emotional disturbances and conflicts appears to an increased number of accidents producing bruises and broken bones.

<u>Death:</u> Death may occur following any of diseases, including the diseases of adaptation mentioned earlier. Alexander (1950) contends that some of these stress-related diseases (I. e: cardiovascular and cancer, etc.) are among the leading causes of death in the United States. Pettelier (1977) maintains that the evidence appears overwhelming for the stress-related nature of the conditions predisposing to fatal heart attack.

Almost any type of traumatic event may trigger the conditions leading to suicide or psychogenic death. The sudden disruptions of an intimate physical relationship, for example, the death of a spouse, a divorce or separation, the breaking of an engagement, the loss of a job, retirement may cause any of a variety of somatic, psychological or emotional disorders which lead to sudden death. In most instances, there is no other apparent reason for the death. Events involving rapid or danger, struggle, or attack produce deaths which we usually attribute to "shock". A variety of types of losses of status or material possessions and failures or defeats, disappointments, and humiliations also may often result in psychogenic death. Engel (1977) contends that even otherwise disposed events (unexpected triumphs, reunions, public recognition, etc) may cause similar results, He also suggests that the normal reciprocity of the fight or flight response may break down under either acute or conflicting stimulations, producing the same results, even small uncertainties may cause momentary cessation of motor activity and cardiac deceleration due to the secretion of certain hormones during the stress reaction.

A number of studies have linked suicide and its resultant condition of depression. Many popular accounts of individual suicides trace them directly to specific traumatic events occurring just before the suicide. Paykel (1976) suggests that depressives accumulate more life change units than other individuals, but those who attempt suicide have the most.

Lowered Effectiveness and Efficiency

There is lack of empirical studies in this area. However, I feel safe in joining other writers on the subject in asserting, on an intuitive basis, some correcting between the factor of impaired effectiveness and expertise and some of the anxiety producing elements of modern life. Generally, one effectiveness and efficiency on the job are usually, higher when we are 'up" than when we are "down". Distress of any kind—mental or physical tends to be distracting. Of course, there are exceptions.

Those who are prone to accidents are obviously, less effective and efficient when their labors are often interrupted by accidents. Reeling of guilt, fear and anxiety interfere with efficiency by diversion one's attention to matters other than work. The depressed individual, obsessed with a sense of helplessness, hopelessness, and possible suicide is highly likely to be much less valuable than the person who can keep his or her thoughts on his or her work. Death, of course is likely to be severely disruptive.

<u>Turnover:</u> Flowers (1975) identifies stress as a significant, if not leading, factor in the causes of executive turnover. In many instances, departures are voluntary, an attempt to escape from stressful situations. In other instances, the exists are stimulated by the employing organization getting rid of deadwood, employees whose performance has been impaired by some of the mediate effects of stress.

<u>Non-turnover:</u> It has been mentioned elsewhere in this book that stress may lead to contrary responses in different individuals, or in the same person at different times. The same kind and level of difficulty which leads one person to leave the organization (the flight) reaction may cause immobility in another. Overwhelmed by fear and anxiety, one may adhere to one's career as the only safe refuge in a world of diversity. Likewise, one's bosses may be incapable of decisive action regarding one's tenure because of their own feelings of fear, guilt, or anxiety. Firing subordinates may be seen as a reflection on their own competence in personnel selection. The net result; lowered productivity for the whole organization, with an increasing number of dropouts. All of the above mentioned mediate effects of stress lead to increased costs of operation to the employing situation.

Summary

In summary, the author concludes that stress is a state of the body manifested by a general adaptation syndrome (G.A.S.). The stress response, the G.A.S is essentially a defense mechanism of the human body, a way of coping with stimuli which threaten either the provision of security (homeostasis) or the preservation of life. It is a extremely difficult process involving, in one way or another, every part of the body in a series of interactions, many of which are, as yet, but dimly understood at the micro level of resolution. The basic pattern of the response is always the same, although there are wide variations in intensity of reactivity, depending upon the individual, cultural and environmental differences, as well as upon the number and duration of exposures to a particular stressor and to stress in general.

As a defense mechanism, the G.A.S is beneficial; it prepares the body for flight or fight in emergency situations, thus tending to ensure self preservation as well as stimulating the self-system to higher levels of performance in demanding situations. It must be noted, however, that, even though it is essentially a defense mechanism, the G.A.S places such severe demands on the body. Each incident of stress level leaves some permanent indication of damage, and these scars accumulate over time to constitute the process of aging. The accumulation of unwanted by products of stress induced chemical reactions in the tissues of the body, and the cumulative effects of continuing loss of body cells (particularly in the brain and heart) constitute the process of exhaustion, the inability to adapt. Thus, the process of aging is, in effect, the gradual exhaustion of the body's resources through the cumulative effects of irreversible wear and tear on the tissues. Further, severe or repeated stress has significant adverse effects of a widely varying nature on the human body and accelerates the depletion of body resources, diminishes the ability to adapt, and speeds the process of aging.

These adverse effects take the form of diseases of adaptation; they occur mainly from improper or inadequate responses by the self-system to stressful stimuli. Of course, some stressors, such as x-rays, extremes of temperatures, severe physical blows, and certain microbes, cause disease regardless of the response. Generally, however, the disease is the result of interaction between the stressor and the self-system. Thus, in addition to the direct effect, of the stressor on the body there are the defensive and defense-inhibiting responses of the self-system. The interactions of these three factors in proper proportions provide the necessary stability for resistance and adaptation of the self-system to the stressor.

Not every departure from homeostasis constitutes disease. Disease occur when the adaptive mechanisms fail adequately to counteract the stressor, or when the self-system over reacts. Disease is not a state or condition, but a dynamic clash of the opposing forces of aggression and defense; it is a struggle to maintain or regain the homeostatic balance of the self-system.

Moreover, every deviation from homeostasis does not create stress; rather, every stimulus received by the self-system causes an abnormality of some degree from the normal amount of homeostasis. In contrast, stress is the state manifested by a specific syndrome—the G.A.S.—which consists of all the nonspecifically induced changes in the self-system responding to a specific stressor. It is the common denominator of all the adaptive reactions of the body, because of the alarm signals involved. While it has its own unique form the G.A.S., it has no single cause. Further, while its manifestations change from moment to moment during the three stages of the G.AS, stress exists throughout the process. In fact, not every instance of stress will progress through all the three stages; only the most severe stress progresses to the third stage of exhaustion, or death. In most instances of stress, the G.A.S. progresses through only the first stages, even when it does progress or temporary, it is not necessarily irreversible.

Also in this chapter the author has discussed a still high level of resolution, first identifying what could be characterized as the mediate effects of stress: physical and mental illness, accidents, deaths, lowered effectiveness and efficiency, professional turnover and non-turnover. Finally, I have suggested some lines along which the readers may speculate for themselves about the long range and ultimate effects of stress.

References

1. Selye, Hans. *Stress.* ACTA Medical Publishers, 1950.
2. Selye, Hans. *The Stress of Life.* New York: McGraw-Hill, 1956.
3. Dertalanffy, L. *General System Theory.* New York: George Braziller, 1968.
4. Cox, Tom. *Stress.* Baltimore: University Park Press, 1980.
5. Ibid.
6. Selye, Hans. *Stress.* ACTA Publishers, 1950
7. Selye, Hans. *The Stress or Life.* New York: McGraw-Hill, 1956
8. Alexander, Franz. *Psychosomatic Medicine: Its Principles and Applications.* New York: Norton, 1950.
9. Freedman, A.M. et al. *Modern Synopsis of Comprehensive Textbook of Psychiatry.* Baltimore: Williams and Wilkins, 1972
10. Flack, Frederick F. *The Secret Strength of Depression.* Philadelphia: J.B. Lippincott, 1974.
11. Seligman, Martin E.P. *Helplessness: On Depression, Development and Death.* San Francisco: Freeman, 1975.
12. Dudley, Donald L., and Elton Welke. *How to Survive Being Alive.* Garden City, N.Y.: Doubleday, 1977
13. Ibid.
14. Alexander, Franz. *Psychosomatic Medicine: Its Principles and Application.* New York: Norton, 1950.
15. Pelletier, Kenneth R. *Mind as Healer, Mind as Slayer.* New York: Dell, 1977.
16. Engel, George. "Emotional Stress and sudden Death", *Psychology Today,* Nov., 1977.
17. Paykel, Eugene S. "Life Stresses, Depression and Attempted Suicide", *Journal of Human Stress,* Sept. 1976
18. Flowers, Vincent S., et al. *Managerial Values for Working* New York: Amacom, 1975.

CHAPTER FOUR

STRESS MANAGEMENT AND COUNSELLING

Coping Mechanisms

As Selye (1974) puts it, there is no panacea for stress; this must be clearly understood from the outset. The proceeding chapters suggest to the reader that stress is highly personal in nature; one person's stress is another person's zest, and vice versa.

In view of this basic fact, the existence of a general treatment, or even a general form of treatment, of stress should not be anticipated. Instead, one might expect to find in the literature on stress a wide range of proposed coping mechanisms and purported cures and, in the fact that is exactly what the author found. However, the author was unable to find any systematic review or treatment of such proposals. The author, therefore, intends to take the lead in that direction.

In the first place, the author suggests disposing of a number of non-techniques, of contraindicated coping mechanisms. Many professionals looking for quick relieve from the adverse effects of stress and impatient of any certainly time consuming scientific or systemic approach to the resolution of their problems, will frequently, and illogically, resort to the point of virtually any manner which show promise of alleviation of the immediate symptoms. The same person who would disdainfully reject any such approach to the solution of an organizational problem, will receive any treatment which provides temporary relief, and without regard to the long range consequences to mental or physical well being.

Unfortunately, the integrity and future security of the organization will be guarded zealously by the professional while neglecting or abusing his or her own self-system, failing to recognize the mutual interdependence of the two. Incapable of personal suffering is other than momentary or at most ephemeral, the teacher, or the nurse seeks solace in palliatives, which, in turn, become habit forming and thereby serve as additional sources of stress in a vicious cycle. Alcohol, tobacco, tranquilizers, sedatives, and certain mind altering drugs are among the most popular of such palliatives.

Alcohol

Alcohol may be useful on the treatment of certain diseases and physical conditions. It should be prescribed by a duly licensed physician. It could be harmful or even fatal in cases of heatstroke or snakebite. However, moderate use of alcohol for occasional relaxation, although still somewhat controversial, probably is not unduly harmful. There seems to be little, if any, evidence that alcohol has any long term adverse effects. It is generally agreed by physicians that the digestion of some individuals may be aided by moderate amounts of wine at mealtime.

Although usually considered being a stimulant, alcohol is actually a depressant. While it may seem to relieve fatigue and provide energy, alcohol actually just lowers certain cerebral inhibitions and thereby provides the illusion of discharge from stress, but at the cost of slowing the evaluation process and neural reflexes, and impairing judgment. At the initial stages, alcohol inhibits hypothalamic activity, countering the effect of the general adaptation syndrome (G.A.S.). Continued ingestion, however, begins to dull the senses and leads ultimately to unconsciousness. Addition (alcoholism) usually results from long term use with concomitant hallucinations and often to the mental condition of delirium tremens.

Also, certain nutritional deficiencies lead to alcoholism because alcohol provides sufficient calories to keep the imbiber from becoming hungry, but the calories are empty, the alcoholic fails to obtain needed vitamins, minerals, and other essential nutrients. 'the deficiency diseases affect the brain, the nerves, and liver. There is sound evidence that heavy drinkers are more susceptible to cancer of the mouth than moderate drinkers to teetotalers. Alcoholism also often results in loss of friends, family, and job, and thereby to financial ruin.

Smoking

Smoking and other uses of tobacco occasionally and in small amounts similarly provide a direct stimulating effect upon the mental and bodily powers, but continued use or abuse of larger amounts have a depressant effect. The narcotic effect or tobacco gives a false sense of freedom from stress and often leads to addition. Continued and excessive smoking, particularly of cigarettes, leads to palpitation and irregularity of the heart; occasional giddy spells; sudden attacks of faintness; liability to exhaustion on slight exertion; dyspepsia and peptic ulcers; dimness of vision and impairment of ability to see colors; chronic sore throat and coughing; cancer of the tongue, mouth, throat, lungs, and bladder and cardiovascular diseases.

Tranquilizers

Tranquilizers provide such an extraordinary degree of success in the treatment of certain psychotic disorders. Tranquilizers tend to produce the mental state of calm, peace, and serenity, free from fear, anxiety, and psychomotor agitation, and without clouding consciousness. The term tranquilizer commonly applies to certain drugs, such a chlorpromazine, reserpine, meprobamate, benactyzine and diazepam (valium). Indiscriminate use of these drugs could lead to dangerous side effects as toxic delirium, jaundice, skin eruptions, asthmatic attacks, and significant changes in blood chemistry.

Sedatives

Sedatives (chiefly the barbiturates and bromides) provide beneficial uses in a limited number of instances and under the direction of a qualified physician; however, such drugs have equally serious adverse effects when used inappropriately. Sedatives may be prescribed for insomnia, headaches and other types of pain, stomach disorders, migraine, emotional disturbances and other adverse effects of stress, with beneficial results. However, they are dangerous and may cause unwanted side effects similar to those mentioned above for tranquilizers. The so called "pep pills" (such as caffeine and Benzedrine) have many more limited beneficial effects. Analgesics (pain relievers) of all kinds are drugs of habituation and should be used only under the direction of a physician.

Narcotics

A narcotic may be defined as a drug which possesses addictively, morphine like analgesic and central depressant activity. Morphine and allied drugs such as cocaine, heroin, and marijuana are narcotic; these drugs are dangerous and must be administered under the supervision and supervision of a duly qualified medical practitioner. The relief from stress that they seem to happen is purely illusory.

All of the above mentioned non techniques have one characteristic in common; they are all typical of the ad hoc approach to management; they are suggested by out-molded particular course habits of thinking; they totally ignore the systems implications of professional stress. At best, such measures constitute mere temporary palliatives; they serve only to relieve some of the symptoms of excessive stress; they interfere with any logical approach to a structured treatment program. They are basically flawed, invalid, and unwarranted.

However, there are a number of more acceptable coping, mechanisms aimed at reducing a person's vulnerability to stress, contacting certain kinds of maladaptive behavior, improving, the stressed person's way of dealing with the vagaries of life.

In this chapter, the author intends to identify treatment, and techniques which seem to be most significant in terms of the treatment they have received from serious students and investigators of the subject. My discussion of each coping mechanism will be limited to an explanation of its general nature and its intended effects.

To facilitate the interpretation and analysis of these coping mechanisms I have established his categorization. I shall distribute the proposed mechanisms into six categories; biofeedback techniques, meditation and relaxation techniques, body (physical) therapies, exercise techniques, dietary regimens, and psychological therapies.

Because stress has many sources and affects many aspects of human functioning, management requires a multifaceted approach with consideration being given to the relief of symptoms, to the sources of stress, and to the conditions that may be responsible for reducing a person's capacity to cope with stressors. To deal with each of these aspects, the stress management and counseling programs must by developed with these objectives: (1) to understand the nature of stress; (2) to establish personal stress response; (3) to establish individual sources of stress; (4) to develop a realistic way to deal with sources of stress; (5) and, to employ relaxation techniques as a coping skill to reduce stress and prevent the accumulation of excessive levels of stress. The requirements of the body for health, the stress response and its effects, possible sources of stress, ways of eliminating stress and practice of relaxation provide the main focus for counseling and therapy.

Biofeedback

According to Payne (1972) there are over two thousand feedback systems in the human body. Wiener (1950) maintains that when one of these feedback mechanisms fails to operate the result is incorrect functioning of one or more parts of the sub-system, for example, in such conditions as intention tremor so parkinsonism. However, these faulty feedback mechanisms may involve blood pressure, heart rate, and even the unconscious raising of hairs on the body or the unconscious dilatation of the pupils in the eye, and not limited to intention tremor and Parkinson's disease.

Biofeedback is simply a means of monitoring one or more of physiological functions of the human body with some type of instrumentation and translating the recorded activity into audio or optical signals (negative feedback) which are transmitted directly to the person whose functions are being monitored. The assumption is that, by observing these signals, learn to exercise some degree of control over the particular function being monitored. Just as the mastery of other motor skills, the person makes use of the continuous stream of sensory feedback signals to modify his or her ongoing performance. Experiments have demonstrated that through this means, one may learn to control such processes. Involuntary or autonomic, and beyond direct conscious control are (1) temperature of specific parts of the body (hands, feet, forehead etc); (2) certain brain waves (particularly Alpha); (3) pulse rate; (4) blood pressure, etc.

Biofeedback instruments exist for many body processes; among the popular are the feedback thermometer, the electroencephalograph (EEG), and the heart rate monitor. More extensive types of equipment exist, but these are usually limited to use in clinical laboratories and will not be discussed here.

Meditation and relaxation

The term, meditation is used here in a general sense to include different types of meditative contemplation, including, specifically, Transcendental meditation, the Relaxation Response developed by Herbert Benson as well as other similar techniques.

The word meditation is usually applied to any state of continual reflection upon a word (mantra), prayer, subject or object (mantras). When the reflection is on an object such as a candle flame, a simple circle, or a crucifix, the eyes are open; otherwise the eyes are normally closed. Meditation is not the same as day dreaming. Some forms of meditation require that the individual silently count breaths one on inhale, two on exhale until ten has been reached, whereupon the sequence beings again at one. The mediator begins again at one on then next inhales. Other forms of meditation require personal silence.

Meditation is usually performed in the normal sitting position (specifically with the back straight), although some Eastern forms of meditation require that the practitioner follow a particular posture, such as sitting with crosses legs (the lotus position). Meditation teachers usually recommend that the practice begin in a quite area with soft lightning, although more experienced practitioners are able to meditate even in brightly lighted, noisy rooms. However, this environment is not recommended for best results. The relaxation of the body and mind, and quieting of the nervous system is supposed to give a definite relief from stress, according to Schifrin, (1976).

There are many varieties of relaxation; in fact, the variety is probably endless and I do not intend to discuss them here. Most of the techniques have reached the West from the East, where every Yogi has his yoga and few of them agree. However, some techniques originated in the Western world, and almost every culture and religion has its own brand of meditation.

In spite of the variations, there are certain fundamental similarities; Maisel (1972) maintains. These include (1) adoption of a passive approach to quite repose, with a reduction of physical and mental activity to a minimum and preferably in a tranquil environment; (2) the repetitive use of some sort of mental device, a focusing of the mind on a singularity in the Hindu varieties, a "mantra" (word or thought), or a " mandala" (physical object), with elimination of all distracting thoughts, ideas, feelings, and emotions; and (3) attainment of an altered state of all thought and worldly feelings, in which the self is liberated from the bonds of the physical body as well as the mind. Although some techniques make the choice after the "mantra" or "mandala" a highly ritualistic and spiritual ritual, the initial idea of concentration is mostly insignificant in it and unrelated to the process of meditation. The "mantra" or "mandala" is solely intended as a device for clearing the mind of all other thoughts. The intense concentration clears the minds of all

distractions and tends to promote the inducement of the altered state or consciousness. The achievement of the altered state of consciousness variously described as mystical, enhanced awareness, deeper consciousness, etc.-represents a model to be strived for, but to be obtained only by the most serious mediators and only after long practice.

Relaxation and Cycle Breaking

Relaxation techniques are extremely powerful coping skills which can be utilized to reduce the severity and duration of stress and to prevent the building up of excess stress.

Relaxation can be achieved through a number of mental and physical means depending on personal preferences and the particular situation. Reading, prayer, exercise or use of a systematic relaxation technique may be beneficial during psychotherapy or counseling, clients may be introduced to progressive muscle relaxation, a procedure that involves first tensing and then relaxing individual muscle groups so that one can understand the feeling of relaxation and thus be more easily able to consciously direct muscles to relax as suggested by Richter and Sloan (1979).

Control through progressive relaxation exercise is best achieved through instruction and diligent practice over a period of tine. It might not be possible to provide in depth study of this technique, and many clients may not practice daily as recommended. For this reason, attention could be placed on "cycle breaking". This technique is, in part, a shortened form of progressive relaxation, and although it may not be as effective, it does seem to have some impact on the level of stress. The main purpose of this technique is to prevent the accumulation of stress by stimulating knowledge or regular assessment of the level of stress in the body and by interjecting small but frequent, measures of relaxation. The activities of "cycle breaking can be extremely circumspect, and it can take as little time as few second to a few minute Clients may be instructed to proceed through the following sequence six times daily, or ideally, every hour.

"Cycle-breaking" can assist the body to become aware of feelings of stress so that he or she can react before the stress becomes severe. According to Mitchell (1977) clients had reported increased awareness of when some effort was required or when a longer "break" was needed to control the intensity and duration of stress.

Stress is a fundamental part of the lives of every individual.

However, too much stress can not only be annoying, but harmful to the physiological, psychological and social aspects of one's existence. By teaching stress management techniques, individuals can achieve greater control of their bodies and move toward an optimal level of health. Other forms of relaxation techniques include Transcendental Meditation, Ethnocentric Meditation, Autogenic Training Progressive Relaxation, Self-directed Relaxation and Breathing.

Stress reduction is perhaps the most emphasized benefit claim of transcendental meditation, and it is this aspect that interests the therapist or the counseling psychologist. According to Kory (1976) even the detractors of transcendental mediation agree that there are a number of benefits that derive from it, even though some of these benefits may be difficult to justify. For example, one benefit often claimed by practitioners has been improved performance at work or in school, together with a greater degree of emotional stability and overall calmness. The relaxed atmosphere and emotional stability, of course, serve as an antidote to stress. Wallace and Benson (1972), in physiological tests observed that experienced mediators approached and crossed the alpha-theta brain wave threshold, a significant indicator of relaxation and calmness. Other techniques such as Zen and Yoga also trigger this relaxation response to emotional changes.

There are several hypotheses to account for the effect of transcendental meditation on the alpha waves, but not much in the process of supporting basic research. There are, however, adequate research funding for the claimed effects on blood pressure, heart rate, metabolic rate, and oxygen consumption. There is, also clinical evidence, in the type of tests of spontaneous skin resistance response, indicating greater stability in the autonomic nervous system on the part of subjects practicing transcendental meditation, even after the meditation. This is indicative of a greater resistance to environmental stress, psychosomatic disease, and performance of the nervous system, Clymes (19770 maintains. There are other forms of relaxation techniques, which I do, not intend to explore in this book.

BODY THERAPY

In this section, I plan to assess four therapies Bioenergetics, Structural Integration,—Awareness through Movement and Structural Patterning—all aimed at correction of the bodily symptoms of stress.

Bioenergetics

Bioenergetics is a neo-Reichian method of psycho—analysis. It combines traditional analysis with body therapy. Kovel (1976) maintains that bioenergetics is essentially Reichian treatment without the forgone hypothesis.

One of the fundamental aspects of bioenergetics is "grounding". Grounding of an electrical circuit is used to as an analogy to illustrate the concept; it is one of the two basic processes of the body: charging up and discharging over. These two processes are generally in balance. Lowen (1972) states that the upper part of the body is primarily concerned with charging up intake of energy (food, oxygen, sensory stimulation). The lower part of the body is primarily concerned with the discharge process through an activity or sexual activity, the experience of pleasure.

Lewen (1972) describes a number of bioenergetics grounding exercise (actually "positions" would be a better communication in view of the connotations of action brought to mind with the term exercise.) One of the positions utilized to develop grounding is to stand with bare feet six inches apart with weight is maintained on the feet. The body should be straight with hands handing loose at the sides. Next the knees are bent, but weight is maintained on the feet. This position should be maintained for two minutes if possible.

The purpose of this position is to bring the patient back in touch with his legs and feet.

Another grounding exercise starts with the feet placed eight inches apart with toes pointed inward. The patient then bends over with knees flexed and touches the ground with his finger tips. Then the patient attempts to straighten the knees until a vibration occurs. The legs should never stiffen nor should the knees be fully extended. Both of these exercises, according to Lowen, will improve circulation or the hands and feet and will increase breathing. There are a number of other grounding exercises, of course, but these two will serve as examples.

Grounding is also used to identify the condition of the patient. Grounding exercise tends to show signs that the therapist can explain. Generally speaking, the patient is clothed in such way as to make these signs more apparent (e.g. leotards or briefs are often used).

In addition to grounding exercises, other exercises are used in the course of therapy. These exercises are called dynamic to distinguish them from the positions described above, for example, lying on the bed and kicking or pinching a bed with fists (women use a tennis racket). This allows the patient to release their anger, the theory being that every patient has something to be passionate about. In bioenergetics treatment about half of the time so spent on body work, the other half of time on traditional psychoanalytic therapy. This division distinguishes it from structural integration.

Structural Integration

Structural Integration is commonly known as Rolfing, after Ida Rolf, who developed this type of therapy. It is designed to elicit a series of orderly changes in the body as a whole. Hamman (1972) sees the lack of stress as the balance of the body within the field in gravity; stress is variation, visible as the inappropriate position of the body components in space.

Structural integration aims to align the body in the gravitational field. A great deal of emphasis is placed in the physical body form and gravity in the Structural Integration studies. According to Dobel (1970, unless the body is properly aligned in relation to gravity there is the possibility that this force may function entropically, disordering and breaking down the body. A basic premise of structural integration is that man is plastic structure and causable of substantial reorganization and change.

In Structural Integration, the body is seen as a tower of blocks in a three dimensional space. The blocks (such as children's building blocks) correspond to head, the thorax, the pelvis, and legs. The way of living and interacting with the environment tends to move these blocks out of perfect alignment. These departures from perfect alignment are seen as deviations which produce compensatory adjustments and strains on other parts of the body. The systems theory concept of moral interconnectivity of subsystems has particular relevance to this line of thought.

Structural integration is essentially a means of applying mechanical energy to manipulate connective tissues, reorganize muscle relationships, and balance the body according to a presumed anatomical structure. This process takes place in a series of ten one –hour sessions which are aimed at sequentially unwinding and freeing the muscles, "decompensation previous compensations", and integrating the entire structure. Rolfers attempt to explore the body as a whole, with emphasis on integrating and rotation the segments, rather than on treating localized symptoms or complaints. The theory behind the manipulation is that the musculature of the body contains memories of psychic traumas that cause the body's disintegration. This is consistent with Powers' view that memory is stored throughout the body. The Rolfer aims to release these memories, and, as a result, the tensions in the rest of the body disappear spontaneously.

Awareness through Movement

According to Reldenkrais (1949) awareness through movement is a set of systematic, slow, gentle exercises based on reversed pattern. A reversed pattern breaks the incessant motion or muscles on the standard gravitational field. The reversed pattern is designed to break up the habituated system of muscles operating under gravitational force. Gravity is minimized by lying on the floor. The exercises emphasize sensing, designed to promote awareness of the body and its movement.

Structural Patterning

This technique is closely associated with the Rolfing movement. It was developed by Judith Aston after taking Rolfing training. All partners, at the minimum, attend the Structural Integration classes before attending Structural Patterning courses. There is hardly any documentation available on Structural patterning, but it is a central core exercise in deep breathing and posture improvement: sitting, standing, walking, etc. Beyond the basic core, Patterning extends into the person's daily activities such as running to ensure that proper posture so being maintained.

Exercise:

Exercise is the single best thing one can do to keep young, according to Dr Hardin B. Jones. And one is never too old to swim or run. Dr. Paul Hutinger says swimming is the closest thing to anti-aging pill. By regularly training older swimmers, he was able to enable them to develop physical abilities of amateur individual 20 to 30 years younger.

Swedish exercise expert and physiologist, Per-Olaf Astrand, also advocates running for good health. In fact, he contends that it is possible to move one's exercise capacity back 15 to 25 years toward birth by a program of heavy training. There is also an added benefit to exercising. Serious exercise can actually increase bone mineral content and strengthen bones beyond the normal limit However, exercise as a technique of combating stress seems controversial. Steincrohn (1973) and other experts believe that exercise is not a means of reducing stress. Other experts disagree. Steincrohn suggests that the rocking chair or hammock will do one more good on weekends than enforced exertion that is anathema to the person.

Friedman (1974) and some other physicians claim that the reward for jogging is a heart attack or death. Light exercise is seems to be of no particular advantage. However, men with lifelong strenuous exercise habits happen to have heart disease at a rate of one-third of other men, Dr Schiemann (1974) suggested.

Pickens (1965) warns against isometric forms of exercise. He defines the term "isometric" as simply pushing, pulling, or lifting against and immovable object by exerting maximum force for a few seconds. The object can be part of one's own body or something steady, such as a post or doorway. He admits that isometric forms of exercise may help a person to develop immense strength and some body tone.

Most experts on the subject of exercise, tend to agree that the best exercises are running, swimming, cycling, and walking, but certainly for those over forty, only with the advice of a physician. It is quite essential for everyone who is about to embark on a vigorous exercise program that they consult with their physicians. Please NOTE that this is not a trivial warning.

One of the few scientific approaches to the prescription of exercise program is that developed by Dr. Kenneth Cooper. He referred to this form of exercise program as "Aerobics" since it is based on the measurement of oxygen consumption. The program is designed so that one may test oneself, determine how much exercise one may want, choose one's own exercise program, and evaluate one's week-to-week progress on a point scale. Those types of exercise recommended include such everyday activities as walking, running, cycling, swimming and a few groups of sports.

Arguably, some exercises are good for us, and some are harmful for us. Exercise that is good for us may depend on the physical and physiological condition of the individual but also on which expert or advocate one consults. There appears to be a dispute or disagreement about exercise, including whether one should indulge in exercise at all. Nevertheless, there is sufficient evidence to suggest that vigorous exercise for someone in good physical condition does not tend to reduce stress and facilitate turning off the emergency response resulting from stress. Once again, the individual is advised to consult a physician in any circumstances.

Diet:

Good nutrition is essential for good health. It is believed that one of the secrets of longevity is learning to choose foods that are good for you, according to Gaylord Hauser. Hauser believes that adding one pint or two cups of freshly made fresh fruit or vegetable juice to your diet daily is one of the best safeguards against pre-mature aging and disease. In addition, Hauser also strongly advocates the use of brewer's yeast, which is essential for our bodies due to its nucleic acids and vitamin B content, which erases facial wrinkles. He recommends brewer's yeast as a life-saving protein that is excellent fortifier of those who cannot afford the expensive forms of protein food.

Dr. Lillian Troll maintains that sufficient protein is an essential. He argues that protein deficiency after age 50 can cause weight loss, fatigue, and premature old age, as the body responds to consuming its protein reserve and loses valuable muscle. Dr. Tomotari suggests that some substance in yogurt may be capable of lowering the amount of cholesterol in the blood, which in turn may help ward off the development of atherosclerotic heart disease. It is advised that out of every 100 grams of protein consumed, only half should be provided by pork or beef. Sweet acidophilus milk is also strongly recommended.

Brown Landons and other longevity researchers believe that sprouts every day keep old age away. They believe that youth-growing substance from new growing sprouts will create cells to grow young. This is because it contains a vital enzyme-like substance known as "axiom". Nutrition experts believe Vitamin C miraculous in its ability to increase one's life span. Eight to 10 grams of ascorbic acid (Vitamin D) daily may extend the life span to 24 years. Nobel Laureate scientist Dr. Linus Pauling says that Vitamin C is fundamentally necessary for every cell in the body, and we do not produce enough of it. Thus, any addition is all to the good.

Other valuable vitamins in stopping the biological clock are Vitamin D and Vitamin B5. More Vitamin D such as those found in fish oils, cod oil, milk, vegetables and seaweed may mean less osteoporosis. It is estimated that about 25 percent of all women past 65 years of age suffer from this condition, which involves demineralization of bones, leaving them porous, fragile and easily broken.

Vitamin B5 is prevalent in protein-rich foods as brewers' yeast, nuts, liver and whole grain cereals and bread. Pantothenic acid (vitamin B5) promotes good health and longevity. Vitamin E is another anti-aging studied. Dr. Cheraskin found that a higher intake of Vitamin E resulted in remarkable of health. Another good rejuvenating element is Propolis, made by bees from tree resins and found in pollen-related products like honey. Dr. John Diamond suggested that Propolis is the most powerful natural stimulant known for thyroid gland health and activity. The thymus governs the body's immune system, and when the thymus is weakened, chronic degenerative disease is able to occur. Propolis is also a powerful antibiotic and is remarkably effective against drug-resistant staphylococcus infections.

Also, it is advisable to go easy on caffeine in one's daily diet. Large amounts of caffeine, in found tea and coffee, tend to remove B vitamins; and B vitamins are vital in maintaining hair color.

Dr. Samuel D. Bonney suggests that one of the easiest ways to prolong your life is to drink plenty of water. Failure to drink enough water can lead to dehydration, which causes damage to the heart and kidneys, and which is responsible for lowering resistance to disease. Arthur Fresse points out that kidney action is reduced by a third between the ages of 20 and 80. Therefore, it is necessary to drink up to eight glasses of water daily. He also advises a minimum intake of salt——— less than 5 grams a day. This is because the sodium compound, salt forces the kidney to work harder than necessary and may increase damage to the liver, probably resulting in hypertension. This is extremely dangerous to people over 55 years of age.

In terms of food consumption, less is better than more as one age; for one calorific needs decline 5 to 10 percent each decade after 20. Women who look younger than their years eat fewer calories, consume considerably less fatty foods of all types and take more Vitamin B1, A and C than those who look older. This based on over 30 years of research by Dr. Schlenker and colleagues.

PSYCHOLOGICAL THERAPIES

Some psychological theories are of the position that individuals, even without training in psychology, can quickly gain insights into their own feelings and behavior, and perhaps, those of others. It is believed that with this insight, one may be able to cope with and possibly eliminate significant stresses in one's life. There are four psycho-therapeutic techniques, namely: Transactional Analysis, Rational-Emotive Therapy, Reality Therapy and Assertive Therapy which may help individual cope with stresses in his life according to the advocates of these theories. The author takes those schools of thought that: (1) are reasonable, rather than highly imaginative, in their approach; (2) can be described simply; and (3) are relatable to stress research.

Transactional Analysis

Transactional Analysis (TA) is one school of thought that meets the above mentioned criteria. It is a way of classification therapy originated by Berne (1964). Transactional analysis postulates that the fundamental unit of social action is a "stroke". Stroking in Transactional Analysis is the psychological equivalent of physical caressing; and it implies recognition. The exchange of strokes is transaction". A casual meeting is a single stroke. Most of individual's social exchanges are so structured that they border on rituals, governed by specific unspoken rules. Generally, these rules remain hidden until an infraction occurs. This gives results in symbolic, verbal, or legal cry of foul.

Transactional Analysis is premised on the hypothesis that each of us has three fundamental psychological ego states. These ego states are not just roles that are being played; they are actually, psychological realities. The three ego states are exteropsychic, which resembles that of a parental figure; (2) neopsychic, which is autonomously directed toward a more nearly objective appraisal of reality and; (3) the archeopsychic, which is dominated by feelings and perspectives fixated in early childhood. The three are more commonly referred to as Parent, Adult, and Child respectively.

The Parent state is characterized by a large collection of recordings assimilated, for the most part, during the first five years of life, and consisting mainly of certain unquestioned basic rules of behavior taught us by one's parents or other authority figures. The Parent state is a necessary and useful part of life; the recorded rules constitute the mores and generally accepted patterns of habit and behavior response to most of the social events in a given culture. The Parent state obviates a lot of unnecessary thinking and decision making in a number of social situations; its existence means, especially that the individual has been programmed to respond in socially acceptable ways.

The Child state is characterized by a series of recorded feelings, assimilated during the early years of life. These recordings are mainly of internal events, the response of the child to what he or she sees, and hears during those early years of life. Harris (1967) argues that most of these recordings are emotional responses, or reflections of the child's inherent dependence, weakness, ineptness and clumsiness.

On the contrary, the Adult state is characterized by mature, discriminatory approach to social transactions. The Adult state is aimed primarily at determining the information value of stimuli, processing and filing the results of such analysis and responding to stimuli on the basis of informed judgments rather than on preprogrammed basis.

Each person integrates these three states in one of an unlimited variety of propositions. Adult state may draw upon both Parent and Child states for information, in addition to its own internalized, data bank. Each person makes a decision and probability estimates with one of the three states having a controlling influence. The propositions are not fixed; they may change from time to time and are subject to conscious influence. For the purpose of coping with stress in one's daily life, Transactional Analysis is one psycho-therapeutic technique which those in need of professional help should at least consider as holding some promise of success in aiding them to improve their interpersonal relations.

Rational Emotive Therapy

The principles and techniques of Rational Emotive Therapy was developed by Dr Albert Allis and expounded by Dr. Robert Harper (1975). Ellis and Harper suggest that some of us allow certain powerful ridiculous and ideological ideas to interfere with us. As a basis Rational Emotive Therapy, Ellis and Harper (1975) provided a list of ten of those irrational ideas. For example, one item on the above-mentioned list suggests (irrationality) that people and things should turn out better than they do, and that must be viewed as awful and terrible if we do not find good solutions to life's harsh realities. But the truth is, of course that there is no reason things should turn out better than they do. Maultsby (1974) argues that everything is exactly the way it should be. His theory is that going back into antiquity the prerequisites for a given reality have been fulfilled in order for any given reality to exist.

To those who complain that people should not behave the way they do, Rational Emotive Therapy (RET) responds that words like, should, ought, must, and their negative equivalents are confused with people desires. RET proponents will say that the preferable way to phrase a harsh reality is to say, "I would have liked it to turn out differently".

RET therapists are of the opinion that if other people behave other than the way we want, we are not adversely affected unless we think it does. RET holds that nobody can make us do anything we do not want to do and that includes feeling bad——no one can feel anything. Lazarus and Fay (1975) went on to say that only the individual can make himself or herself feel depressed or content or experience any other emotion.

It would seem that RET gives the individual some insight into many facets of stress. How much stress is due to unreasonable ideas of what "should" be? Besides, how much stress is caused by our ridiculous expectations of other's behavior? One way to find out is to monitor one's internal dialogue, according to Goodman and Maultsby. Call this "self-talk".

It should be pointed out that behavior and emotions do not just happen in the brain. These emotions and behaviors have thought content, and regularly take the form of conversations. We will be able to analyze this dialogue for its practical content, we write it down. However, Goodman and Maultsby points out that when individuals or patients are first going through the process of learning to isolate and articulate their irrational self-talk is when they are in the most need of professional guidance, or at least experienced advice from ex-patients. For a relatively healthy, even though stressed person, guidance in identifying self-talk is probably not necessary, although at first, such analysis may be difficult. However, gaining some insight into what one is saying to oneself is positive.

Reality Therapy

Reality Therapy was proposed by William Glasser (1965). The basic tenet of Reality Therapy is that individuals must accept responsibility for their own actions and behavior. Reality Therapy does not accept the idea of mental illness, nor does it accept the premise that current behavior is the result of the past.

The author has included Reality Therapy here due to the fact that among the prevailing types of psychotherapy, Reality Therapy takes cognizance of changes that are taking place in society. Glasser (1965) asserts that while the institutions of North American (and possibly other societies also) act as if goal takes precedence over the role, the fact remains that role, or identity appears to be now so important that it must be achieved before we found out to find a goal. Glasser's position is consistent the opinion of Graves and others that evolution in the level of psychological existence is taking place.

For the individual, the significance of Glasser's theory lies in relevance to his or her interpersonal relations, especially his or her other relationships with other people who are seeking identity or role rather than the traditional goals of society. Unlike other traditional forms of therapy, individuals engaged in Reality Therapy are encouraged to discuss current events, not the past. By pointing out the differences between responsible and irresponsible behavior, the therapists attempt to get the client to see how he or she is currently acting. Irresponsible behavior is not excused by the therapist on the grounds of negative emotions, e.g. anger, feeling rejected or hurt, etc.

Assertive Therapy

Assertive Therapy is referred to under a variety of names, such as assertiveness training and assertive behavior. Essentially it identifies three basic types of behavior: non-assertive, assertive, and aggressive. Aggressive behavior is seen when as behavior when that results in "put down" another person. Non-assertive behavior results when individuals are denying themselves or inhibited from expressing their feelings, perhaps because they are polite. Alberti and Emmons (1975) describe assertive behavior as that behavior which results from choice and results in individuals feeling good.

There seem to be two reasons why a person could be involved in assertive training. The first reason is that one can expect people to become assertive and refuse to be manipulated. Unfortunately, not only they are being trained to defend themselves, but the finishing touch on most of their authoritative statements tends to be obnoxious.

Assertive therapy attempts to get people to focus on interpersonal relationships and goals. The Assertive therapist encourages his or her patients to monitor their own behavior and especially keep track of the number of times they have been assertive. Written homework is stressed in order to keep track of progress. Behavior modification techniques are used as imagining situations which trigger anxiety or aggressive behavior, the client imagines ways of dealing with the imagined situation in an assertive way. The individual is then encouraged to practice assertive behavior in similar real-life situations.

Relationship of Coping Mechanisms to Causes of Stress

The preceding discussion identifies the basic mechanisms proposed in the literature for coping with stress. As indicated, there are wide varieties of other techniques, most of which are simply variations or modifications of those discussed earlier. Some are highly touted as cure-alls others make more modest claims. Almost all, however, claim some benefits in the way or providing general relief from symptoms of stress.

An analysis of each of the proposed coping mechanisms, however, one finds that the technique is usually more specific in its application, being directed at the alleviation or elimination of one or more of the physiological and/ or psychological causes of stress. The author leaves to each person the task of determining for himself or herself the value of each these coping mechanisms in consultation with his or her psychiatrist, psychologist or mental health counselor.

Coping Mechanisms and the Physiological Causes of Stress.

So far, the write has no coping mechanisms specifically directed as to the causes identified as a genetic trait and inherent problems. However, there are four types of techniques aimed at correction of dysfunctional biological rhythms: biofeedback, meditation and relaxation, body therapy and exercise. Only one method is directed to sleeplessness: biofeedback. For the correction of dietary deficiencies a plethora or suggestions contained in the literature, almost all of which are highly controversial, involving, as they do, either greater reliance on, or the complete elimination of, one or more of the generally accepted articles of the typical Canadian or American diet.

At least for techniques make some claim, more or less acceptable, for relief or cure of one or more diseases: biofeedback (migraine, hypertension), meditation and relaxation (hypertension), exercises (heart and lung ailments; diet (migraine and a variety of disease conditions). Body treatment and exercise routines are directed at correction of improper posture and diseases and conditions resulting there from. Four of the listed techniques aimed at alleviation of muscular tension and fatigue: biofeedback, meditation, and relaxation, body therapy and exercise.

Coping Mechanisms and the Psychological Causes of Stress

Comparing the list of psychological causes of stress, it seems that there are only four psychological therapies with any general relaxation applicability. In addition, biofeedback, meditation-relaxation, and body therapy claim some benefits in the relief of anxiety. Meditation and relaxation techniques also apply to failure.

Also, biofeedback influences both perceptions and feelings and emotions. Meditation and relaxation techniques influence perceptions, feelings and emotions, perception, life experiences, life situations, life decisions and behavior. Of course, all the therapies mentioned influence behavior through their effects on the elements of self-esteem.

Coping Mechanisms and the Environmental Causes of Stress

In view of the fact that all of the proposed coping mechanisms are directed at the internal operations of the human body—physical and mental—they obviously have no direct applicability to the management of external stressors. Instead, they aim to improve the individual's ability to cope with, at least certain, external stressors.

Summary

As with the causes of stress, there appears to be no systematic treatment of the remedies of stress currently available, much less any proposals for a systematic approach to the management of stress. For the most part, the coping mechanisms in the literature appear to be techniques for relieving accumulated stress or for offsetting some of its adverse effects. The application of these techniques is analogous to ad hoc approach to management, such as applying grease to the squeaking wheel.

Medication can cause a calming effect on the individual and will this, at least have short term beneficial effects. Probably the most salient aspects of approaches have been discussed are their applicability to learning theory. The common thread running through these approaches is that the individual can learn specific techniques, which will allow him or her to handle, or at least cope with, the stresses of life.

Of the four psychological therapies earlier described, two—Transactional Analysis and Rational Emotive Therapy—would seem to be most beneficial to first review or examine. However, any of these techniques may provide some insight into the way people think and behave and the purpose thereof. Of course, there is nothing magic about the four techniques I have discussed. For information that may lead to improved self-understanding and stress reduction, the field of psychology offers numerous possibilities.

References

1. Selye, Hans, *Stress without Distress*. Philadelphia: Lippincott, 1974.
2. Cox, Tom, *Stress*. Baltimore: University Park Press, 1980.
3. Goodman
4. Cox, Tom, *Stress*. Baltimore: University Park Press, 1980
5. Payne, Buryl, *Getting There Without Drugs*. New York
6. Wiener, Norbert. *The Human Use of Human Beings: Cybernetic and Society*. New York: Avon, 1950
7. Shiffrin, Nancy, *Encounter: A Guide To New Low Cost Techniques*. Chatsworth, Calif.: Major Brooks, 1976.
8. Maisel, Edward. *Tai Chi for Health*. New York: Holtm Rinehart & Winston, 1972.
9. Ibid.
10. Richter, Judith, and Sloan, Rebecca. "Stress: A Relaxation Technique", *American Journal of Nursing*. 79: 1960-1964, Nov. 1979.
11. Mitchell, Laura. *Simple Relaxation*. London: John Murray, 1977, p.126.
12. Kory, Robert B. *The Transcendental Meditation Program for Business People*. New York: Amacom, 1976.
13. Wallace, Robert K., and Hubert Benson, "The Psychology of Meditation", *Scientific American*, 226:2, 80-90, 1972.
14. Clymes, Manfred. *Sentics: The Touch of Emotions*. Garden City, N.Y.: Doubleday Anchor Books, 1977.
15. Kovel, Joe. *A Complete Guide to Therapy*. New York: Pantheon, 1976
16. Haaman, Kalen, "What Structural (Rolfing) Is and Why It Works", *The Osteopathic Physician*, March 1972.
17. Sobel, David S. "Gravity and Structural Integration" in Robert E. Ornstein (Ed), *The Nature of Human Consciousness*. San Francisco, Calif. Freeman Press, 1973.
18. Feldenkrais, M. *Body and Mature Behavior*. New York: International University Press, 1949.

19. Steincrohn Peter J. *Questions and Answers about Nerves, Tension and Fatigue.* New York: Hawthorn, 1973.
20. Friedman, Meyer and R.H. Roseman. *Type of Behavior and Your Heart.* New York: Knopf, 1974.
21. Sheimann, Eugene. *Sex Can Save Your Heart and Life.* New York: Bantom, 1974.
22. Pickens, R.E. *The NLF Guide to Physical Fitness.* New York: Random House, 1965.
23. Miller, Benjamin F. et al. *Free from Heart Attacks.* New York: Simon & Schuster, 1972.
24. Goulart, Francis Sheridan. *Eat to Win Food Psyching for Athlete.*
25. Berne, Eric, *The Structure and Dynamics of Organizations and Groups.* New York: Grove Press, 1963.
26. Harris, Thomas A. *I'M OK—You're OK: A Practical Guide to Transactional Analysis.* New York: Harper & Row, 1967
27. Mok, Paul P. *Transactional Analysis Tool Kit.* Dallas, Texas: Transactional Analysis Press, 1975.
28. Ellis, Albert and R.A. Harper. *A New Guide to Rational Living.* Eglewood Clifs, N.H: Prentice-Hall, 1975.
29. Lazarus, Arnold and Allen Fay. *I Can If I Want To.* New York: William Morrow, 1975
30. Glasser, William. *Reality Therapy: A New Approach to Psychiatry.* New York: Harper & Row, 1965
31. Albertini, R.E., and M.L. Emmons. *Stand Up, Speak Out And Talk Back: The Key to Self-Assertive Behavior.* New York: Pocket Books, 1975.

CHAPTER FIVE

STRESS MANAGEMENT TECHNIQUES IN OTHER CULTURES AND RELIGIONS

In this chapter, the writer will discuss stress management techniques cross culturally and in other religions. The various techniques of meditation used to manage stress cross-culturally can be classified. Some focus on the field or background knowledge and experience also referred to as "mindfulness"; others focus on preselected specific goal, and are called "concentrative" meditation. There are also techniques that shift between the field and the goal.

In "mindfulness meditation", the mediator sits comfortably and quietly, centering attention by focusing awareness on an object or activity such as the breath; a sound-like mantra, visualization or an exercise). The mediator is usually encouraged to keep a clear focus.

Hinduism

Meditation is said to have originated from Vedic Hinduism, which is the oldest religion that professes meditation as a spiritual and religious practice. Evidence as to the origins of meditation extends back to a time before recorded history. Archeologists tell us the practice may have existed among the first Indian civilizations. India scriptures dating back to

5000 years describe meditation techniques. From its early beginnings and over thousands of years, meditation has developed into a structured practice used today by millions of people worldwide of different nationalities and religious background.

Yoga is one of the six schools of Hindu philosophy focusing on meditation (Giri. et al. 2007). In India, yoga is seen as a means to both mental and physiological mastery. There are different types of meditation in Hinduism:

Vadanta: A form of Jnana Yoga

Raja Yoga: This according to Patanjali, describes eight "limbs" of spiritual practices, half of which might be classified as meditation. Underlying them is the notion that a yogi should still be the fluctuations of his or her mind. Surat shabd yoga or "sound and light meditation"

Japa Yoga, in a mantra is repeated aloud or silently. Bhati Yoga, the yoga of love and affection, in which the seeker is focused on an object of devotion, e.g. Krishna.

Hatha Yoga, in which postures and meditations are aimed at raising the spiritual energy, known as "Kundalini", which rises through energy centers known as "chakras"

The objective of meditation is to achieve a relaxed state of mind. Patanjali (1984), in his Yoga Sutras, described five different states of mind: Ksipta; Mudha; Viksipta; Ekagra; and Nirodha. Ksipta defines an agitated mind, unable to determine, attend or keep or remain quite. It is jumping from one thought to another. In Mudha, no information seems to reach the brain; the person is preoccupied. Viksipta is a higher state where the brain receives information, but is unable to process. It moves from one thought to another, in a confused inner speech. Ekagra is a state of a calm mind but not asleep. The person is focused and can pay attention. Finally, Nirodha, when the mind is not disturbed by erratic thoughts; it is totally focused as when one is meditating or totally centered in what one is doing. The ultimate goal of meditation according to

Patanjali (1984) is the destruction of primal ignorance and the relaxation of and establishment in the existential nature of the Self.

Meditation has been stressed by all religions. The meditative state of mind is declared by the Yogis to be the highest state in which the mind exists. When the mind is studying the external object, it gets identified with it, loses itself. To use the simile of the ancient Indian philosopher; the soul of man is like a piece of crystal. But it takes the color of whatever is near it. It is meditation that brings us nearer to the truth than anything else.

Buddhism

Meditation has always been central to Buddhism and considered an essential tool in spiritual development. Most forms of Buddhism distinguish between two classes of meditation practices, sharmatha and vipassana, both of which are necessary for attaining enlightenment. The former consists of training aimed at developing the ability to focus the attention single-pointedly; the latter includes practices aimed at developing understanding and wisdom through seeing the nature of reality. The differentiation between the two types of meditation practices is not always clear cut, which is made apparent when studying practices such as Anapanasti which could be said to start off as a sharmatha practice but goes through a number of stages and end up as a vipassana practice.

Thus, meditation is considered as the way to bring back to oneself, where we can experience and taste one's entire being, beyond all habitual patterns. In the stillness and silence of meditation, we glimpse and return to that deep spiritual nature that we have so long ago lost sight of amid the business and diversion of one's minds. Most Buddhist believes that the gift of learning to meditate is the greatest gift we can give ourselves in this life. For it is only through meditation that we can undertake the journey to discover one's true nature, and so get the strength and trust we will need to live, and die, well. Meditation is the path to enlightenment.

Most Buddhist traditions recognize that the path to Enlightenment entails three types of training: virtue; meditation (Samadhi); and, wisdom (panna). Thus, meditative prowess alone is not sufficient; but it is but one of the paths. In other words, Buddhism, in tandem with mental cultivation, moral development and rational understanding are also needed for the attainment of the highest goal (Western Buddhist Review).

Christianity

Christian traditions have different practices, which can be, identified as a variety of "meditation". Monastic traditions are the basic for many of these practices. Practices such as the rosary, the Adoration (focusing on the Eucharist) in Catholicism or the hesychast practice in Eastern Orthodoxy, may be compared to forms of Eastern meditation that focus on an individual object. Christian meditation is considered a form of prayer. Hesychastic, practice may require recitation of the Jesus prayer, thus through the grace of God and one's own efforts, to concentrate in the heart and mind. Prayer as a form of meditation of the soul is described in the Philokalia—-—a practice that leads towards Theosis which ignores the senses and results in spiritual stillness.

The Old Testament book of Joshua sets out a variety of meditation based on scriptures: "Do not let this Book of the law depart from your mouth, meditate on it day and night, so that you may be prudent to do everything written in it, then one will be prosperous and successful" (Joshua 1:8). This is one of the reasons why Bible verse memory is a tradition among many evangelical Christians (Christian Meditation, 2008).

Islam

Meditation in Islam, Nigosian (2004) maintains, is the basis of its creed. A Muslim is obligated to pray five times a day (before dawn, noon, afternoon, dusk and night). During those times of prayer, the Muslim is expected to focus and meditate on Allah through recitation of AL Qur'an and dhikr in order to build and strengthen the relationship between Allah/Creator and creation. This, in turn, is meant to guide the soul to reality. The meditation is intended to help the Muslim maintain spiritual peace in spite of challenges they may encounter in their work, social and family life. In this manner, the five daily times of peaceful prayer are meant to serve as a model for the Muslim's performance during the whole day, transforming into a single, sustained meditation.

Meditation quiescence is believed to have a quality of healing and creativity. The Muslim prophet Muhammad, whose deeds devout Muslims follow, spent long periods in meditation and contemplation. It was during one such period of meditation that Muhammad began to receive revelations of the Qur'an. The following are two more concepts or schools of meditation in Islam.

Tafakkur and Tadabbur, literally meaning thinking the reflection upon the universe. Muslims believe this is a form of intellectual development which emanates from higher level, i.e. from Allah. This intellectual process through the receiving of divine inspiration awakens and liberates the human mind, permitting man's inner personality to develop and grow so that he may spend his or her life on a spiritual plane far above the mundane level. This is consistent with overall teaching of Islam, which views life as an indication of one tradition of obedience to Allah.

The second type of meditation is the Sufi meditation, which is largely based on religious exercises. However, this method is somewhat controversial among Muslim scholars.

One group of Ulama, Al-Ghazzali, for instance, has accepted it; another group of Ulama, Ibn Taymiya, for instance, have rejected it as a bid'ah (religious innovation).

Jainis

The Jainis use the word Samayika, a word in the Prakrit language from the word samay (time), to denote the practice of meditation. The aim of Samayika is to transcend the everyday experiences of being a "constantly changing" human being. Jiva, allows for the identification with the "changeless" reality in the practitioner, the Atma. The practice of Samayika begins by achieving a balance in time. If the present moment of time is taken to be a point between the past and the future, Samayika means being fully aware, alert and conscious in that very moment, experiencing one's true nature, Atma, which is considered common to all living beings.

Meditation techniques were present in ancient Jain scripture that have been forgotten with time.

Judaism

Shapiro (2007) contends that there is evidence that Judaism has had meditative practices that date back thousands of years. For instance, in the Torah, the Patriarch Isaac described as going "lasuach" in the field, a term understood by all commentators as some sort of meditative practice (Genesis 24:63), probably prayer. Similarly, there are indications throughout the Hebrew Bible that meditation was central to the prophets. In the Old Testament, there are two Hebrew words for meditation, "haga", which means to sigh or moan, but also to meditate, and "siha", which means to recite in one's mind.

In recent Jewish tradition, one of the best known meditative practices is called "hitbodedut", which derives from the Hebrew word "boded", (a state of being alone) and said to be related to the sfirah of Binah, which means the process of making oneself understand a concept well through systematic study.

New Age Meditation

New Age meditations, Tart (1995) argues, are often influenced by Eastern philosophy and mysticism such as Yoga, Hinduism, Buddhism, yet may contain some amount of Western influences. In the west meditation found its mainstream roots through the hippie, counterculture and social transformation of the 1960s and 1970s when many of the youth of the day rebelled against traditional belief systems.

Sikhism

In Sikhism, the practice of simran and Nam Japo encourage quite meditation. This is focusing one's attention on the attributes of God. Sikhs believe that there are ten "gates" to the body. "Gates" is another word for "chakras or energy centers". The top most energy level the tenth gate or dasam dwar. It is believed that when one reaches this stage through continuous practice, meditation becomes a tradition that continues whilst waking, talking, eating, awake, and even sleeping. There is a distinct taste or flavor when a mediator reaches this lofty stage of meditation as one experiences absolute peace and tranquility inside and outside the body.

Taoism

Taoism includes a number of meditative and contemplative traditions. Taoism internal martial arts, especially Tai Chi Chuan were thought of as moving meditation. A common phrase being, "movement in stillness" referring to energetic movement in passive Qigong and seated Taoist meditation, with the converse being "stillness in movement", a state of mental calm and meditation in tai chi form.

Baha'i Faith

According to Smith (1999), the Bahai Faith teaches that meditation is necessary for spiritual growth, alongside obligatory prayer and fasting. The Baha'i Faith holds the view that meditation is the basis for opening the doors of mysteries to our minds. In that state man withdraws himself from all outside objects; in that subjective mood he is immersed in the ocean of spiritual life and can reveal the secrets of things-in-themselves.

Krishnamurti Concept of Meditation

Krishnamurti (1999) used the word meditation to mean something entirely different from the practice of any system or process to control the mind. He said that for people to escape his conflicts has invented many forms of meditation. These have been based on passion, will, and drive for achievement, and imply conflict and a struggle to succeed. This conscious, deliberate striving is always within the limits of a conditioned mind, and in this there is no freedom. All attempts to meditate are the denial of meditation. Meditation is the ending of thought. It is only then there is a different dimension which is beyond measure. Krishnamurti believes that prayer is a choiceless awareness in the present. He argues that when we learn about ourselves, watch ourselves, watch the way we walk, how we eat, what we say, the gossip, the hate, and jealousy—if we are aware of all that in ourselves, without any choice, that is part of meditation.

Active/Dynamic Meditation

Dynamic meditation is the name of one of Osho's popular Active Meditation techniques. However, in general active/

dynamic meditation refers to any meditation technique which does not have one's body assuming a fixed posture. Such techniques are widely used in Karma Yoga.

Osho, earlier introduced the meditation technique which he termed Active Meditations, which begins with dynamic level of activity, sometimes severe and physical, followed by a period of silence. He emphasized that meditation is not concentration. Dynamic meditation involves a conscious catharsis where one can throw out all the repressions, express what is not easily expressible in society, and then easily progress into silence. Some of his techniques also have a stage of spontaneous dance. Osho maintains that if people are innocent there is no need for Dynamic Meditation. But if people are repressed, psychologically, are carrying a lot of a burden, then they need cleansing.

Health Applications of Meditation

The behavioral components of the following meditation techniques are believed by medical scientists to be helpful:

1. Relaxation
2. Concentration
3. Altered state of awareness
4. Suspension of logical thought process, and
5. Maintenance of self-observing attitude.

The medical community has studied the physiological effects of meditation; determine its impact on somatic motor function as well as cardiovascular and respiratory function. Meditation has entered the mainstream of health care as a method of stress and pain reduction. Meares (1976) reported in the "Medical Journal of Australia", the regression of cancer following intensive meditation.

As a method of stress reduction, meditation is often used in hospitals in cases of chronic or terminal illness to reduce complications associated with increased stress including an impaired immune system. There is growing consensus in the medical community that psychological factors such as stress significantly contribute to lack of physical health. Austin (1999) reported that Zen meditation rewires the circuitry of the brain in his landmark book, "Zen and the Brain". This has been confirmed using functional MRI imaging which examines the activity of the brain. Benson (2000), reports that meditation induces a lot of biochemical and physical changes in the body collectively referred to as "relaxation response". The relaxation response includes changes in metabolism, heart rate, respiration, blood pressure and brain chemistry.

WARNING: Readers of this book should not embark upon any of the stress reduction techniques outlined in this book without prior consultation with their physicians and/or qualified mental health professionals.

References

1. Dharmacarini Manishini, *Western Buddhist Review* assessed at: http//www.westernbuddhistreview.com/vol14/kamma-in-context.
2. Smith, P (1999), *A Concise Encyclopedia of the Baha'I Faith,* Oxford, UK: Oneworld Publication, p.243.
3. Shapiro, R (2007) *A Brief Introduction to Jewish Meditation.* www. tripod.com. Retrieved on August 25, 2007.
4. Tart, C. *Adapting Eastern Spiritual Teachings in Western Culture," Journal of Transpersonal Psychology," 22, pp. 149-166.*
5. The World Community for Christian Meditation, www.wccm.org, February 2, 2008.
6. Nigosian, S.A (2004), *Islam, Its History, Teaching and Practices.* Bloomington: Indiana University Press.
7. MirAhmadi, A (2005).*Healing Power of Sufi Meditation.* Publisher: Islam Supreme Council of America.

8. Rincpoche S, *The Tibetan Book of Living and Dying*, ISBN 0-06-250834-2.
9. Sri, N.P (2005), *Meditation is for You: An introduction to the Science and Art of Meditation*, ISBN 8190243748.
10. Austin, James H (1999), *Zen and the Brain: Toward an Understanding of Meditation and Consciousness*. Cambridge: MIT Press.

BIBLIOGRAPHY

Anspaugh D.J et al. (2009) "Coping with and managing stress," in *Wellness Concepts and Applications* 7th ed. Pp 312-329. New York: McGraw-Hill.

Axelrad, A.D, et al. (2009), *Hypnosis*, in B.J.Sadock, et al eds. Comprehensive Textbook of Psychiatry", 9th ed. Vol. 2. pp. 2804-2832. Philadelphia: Lippincott Williams and Wilkins.

Bond M. (1988) *Stress and Self Awareness: A Guide for* Nurses.

Benson, Herbert (1992), *The Relaxation Response*. Harper Collins: New York.

Bower, J.E & Segerstrom S.C. (2004). "*Stress Management, findings, benefits, and immune function: positive mechanisms for intervention effects on physiology*". Journal of Psychosomatic Research 56 (1); 9-11.

Bradley, D. (2000) *Hyperventilation Syndrome*, Kyle Cathie Ltd.

Brookes, D (1997) *Breathe Stress Away*, Hollanden Publishing.

Chaitow, L, et al. (2002) *Multidisciplinary Approaches to Breathing Pattern Disorders*. Churchill Livingstone.

Bull, Steven J. *Sport Psychology—A Self Help Guide*. Crowood Press: Marborough, UK.

Cooper, C.L. et al (1987) *Living with Stress*, Penguin.

Cooper, C.L. *Handbook of Stress Medicine and Health*, CRC Press.

Cooper C., Palmer S (2000) *Conquer Your Stress*, Chartered Institute of Personnel and Development.

Cooper, K. (1991) *Overcoming Hypertension*. Bantam Books.

Craig, Eric, *Stress as a Consequence of the Urban Physical Environment,* in Goldbenger, L. & Breznitz, S, Eds. The Handbook of Stress, Free Press: New York.

David M (2000) *Relaxation and Stress Reduction Work* Book, New Harbinger Inc.

Davis, Martha (2000). *The Relaxation & Stress Reduction Workbook (Fifth Edition).* New Habinger Publications: Oakland, California.

Dimsdale. Et al (2009). "Stress and Psychiatry." In B.J Sadock et al. eds. *Comprehensive Textbook of Psychiatry* 9th ed. Vol.2, pp.2407-2423, Philadelphia: Lippincott Williams and Wilkins

Edwards, M. (2002). *Stress Management for Cancer Patients: A Self Help Manual,* Acorn Publishing.

Elkin, Allen. (2001). *Stress Management for Dummies.* Hungry Minds, New York,

Everly G.S (1989), *A Clinical Guide to the Treatment of the Human Stress Response* sis, Plenum Press.

Fried R (1990). *The Breathe Connection.* Plenum Press.

Fried R (1999) *Breathe Well Be Well,* John Wiley and Sons Inc.

Goldberger, I & Breznit, S. (Eds). 1993. The Handbook of Stress. Free Press: New York.

Green, Don, *Fight Your Fears and Win.* Random House: New York.

Greenberger, Dennis & Christine Padesky (1995), *Mind Over Mood,* The Guildford Press: New York

Hambly K. Muir A. (1997) *Stress Management in Primary Care,* Butterworth Heinemann

Hobfoll, Steven E & Alan Vaux, *Social Support, Resources and Control Context.* "Handbook of Stress". Leo Goldberger & Shlomo Ed. The Free Press: Toronto, Canada.

Hoffman D. (1986) *The Holistic Herbal Way to Successful Stress Control,* Thorsons.

Hoffman, D (1992) *Therapeutic Herbalism*

Howell M, Whitehead J (1989), *Survive Stress: A Training Program*, Cambridge Health Promotion.

Hubbard J.R., Workman E.A (1988), *Handbook of Stress Medicine*, CRC Press.

Jones H (1997), *I am too Busy to be Stressed,* Hodder and Stoughton.

Krista, Alix (1987). *The Book of Stress Survival.* Guild Publishing: London, UK

Lehrer P.M. Woolfolk R.L (2007), *Principles and Practices of Stress Management,* The Guildford Press.

Leonard Brown S (2001), *Stress and Depression.* Hodder.

Mandler, G. "Thought, Memory and Learning Effects of Emotional Stress." *The Handbook of Stress,* Goldberger L, ed. (1993). Free Press, New York

Martin P. (1997) *The Healing Mind: The Visual Link between Brain and Behavior, Immunity and Disease.* Thomas Dunne Books.

Martens, Rainer (1987) *Coaches Guide to Sports Psychology, Human Kinetics.* Champaign: Illinois

Motzer, S.A & Hertig V (2004), *Stress, Stress Response and Health. Nursing Clinics of North America,* 39: 1-17.

Murray, M.T & Pizzorno, J.E (2006), *Stress Management.* In J.E Pizzorno, Jr, M.T. Murray, eds. Textbook of Natural Medicine, 3rd Edition, vol. pp 701—708. St. Loius: Churchill Livingstone.

O'Hara,V (1995). *Wellness at Work,* The New Harbinger Inc.

Palmer S & Dryden W (1995), *Counseling for Stress Problems,* Sage: Columbia.

Payne R (1995), *Relaxation Techniques: A Practical Handbook for Healthcare Professionals,* Churchill Livingstone.

Pines, Ayala M, *Handbook of Stress (1993).* The Free Press: Toronto, Canada.

Posen D (1995), *Stress Management for Physicians and Patient,* Web Article

Powell, T.J. Enright S.J, (1993), *Anxiety and Stress Management*, Routledge.

Seaward B.L (1999), *Managing Stress: Principles and Strategies for Health and Wellbeing*, 2nd edition, Jones and Barlett Publishers.

Steptoe, A (1997). "Stress and Disease." *The Cambridge Handbook of Psychology, Health and Medicine*. Cambridge University Press: Cambridge, UK.

Seymour D.J. & Black K (2002), "Stress in primary care patients." In F.V. DeGruy III et al., ed. *20 Common Problems in Behavioral Health*, pp. 65-87, New York: McGraw-Hill.

Simmons M, Daw W (1994), *Stress, Anxiety, Depression: A Practical Workbook*, Winslow Press.

Spiegel H, et al.(2005) in B.J.Sadock, V.A. Saddock, eds. *Kaplan and Saddock's Comprehensive Textbook of Psychiatry*, 8th ed., vol. 2, pp. 2548—2568. Philadelphia: Lippincott Williams and Wilkins.

Steinmetz J. (1980), *Managing Stress Before It Manages You*, Bull Publishing.

Taylor, S.E (1999), *Health Psychology*. (The Fourth Edition), McGraw-Hill: Singapore

Timmons B.H., Ley R (1994), *Behavioral and Psychological Approaches to Breathing Disorders*, Plenum Press.

Townsend J. (2000), *Get Tough With Stress*.

Trickett M. (2001), *Anxiety and Depression: A Natural Approach*, Ulysses Press.

Tyler M (1999), *Stress Management Training for Trainers Handbook*, Living with Stress Ltd.

Weller S (2000), *The Breath B00k: 20 Ways to Breathe Away Stress, Anxiety and Fatigue*, Thorsons.

White J (1997), *Stress Pac*, The Psychological Corporation.

Wilkinson G (1999), *Family Doctor Guide to Stress*, Dorling Kindersley.

Wolfgang, Linden, et. Al. (2001), "Individualized Stress Management for Primary Hypertension: A Randomized Trial," *Arch Intern Med 161*: 161-1080

Lightning Source UK Ltd.
Milton Keynes UK
UKOW03f1843120314

228051UK00001B/26/P